Leadership, Management and Team Working in Nursing

Transforming Nursing Practice series

Transforming Nursing Practice is the first series of books designed to help students meet the requirements of the NMC Standards and Essential Skills Clusters for degree programmes. Each book addresses a core topic, and together they cover the generic knowledge required for all fields of practice. Accessible and challenging, *Transforming Nursing Practice* helps nursing students prepare for the demands of future healthcare delivery.

Core knowledge titles:

Series editor: Dr Shirley Bach, Head of the School of Nursing and Midwifery at the University of Brighton

Communication and Interpersonal Skills in Nursing (2nd. ed)	ISBN 978 0 85725 449 8
Contexts of Contemporary Nursing (2nd. ed.)	ISBN 978 1 84445 374 0
Health Promotion and Public Health for Nursing Students	ISBN 978 0 85725 437 5
Introduction to Medicines Management in Nursing	ISBN 978 1 84445 845 5
Law and Professional Issues in Nursing (2nd. ed.)	ISBN 978 1 84445 372 6
Leadership, Management and Team Working in Nursing	ISBN 978 0 85725 453 5
Learning Skills for Nursing Students	ISBN 978 1 84445 376 4
Medicines Management in Adult Nursing	ISBN 978 1 84445 842 4
Medicines Management in Children's Nursing	ISBN 978 1 84445 470 9
Medicines Management in Mental Health Nursing	ISBN 978 0 85725 049 0
Nursing Adults with Long Term Conditions	ISBN 978 0 85725 441 2
Nursing and Collaborative Practice (2nd. ed)	ISBN 978 1 84445 373 3
Nursing and Mental Health Care	ISBN 978 1 84445 467 9
Passing Calculations Tests for Nursing Students	ISBN 978 1 84445 471 6
Patient and Carer Participation in Nursing	ISBN 978 0 85725 307 1
Successful Practice Learning for Nursing Students (2nd. ed)	ISBN 978 0 85725 315 6
What is Nursing? Exploring Theory and Practice (2nd. ed.)	ISBN 978 0 85725 445 0

Personal and professional learning skills titles:

Series editors: Dr Mooi Standing, Principal Lecturer/Professional and International Lead in the Department of Nursing and Applied Clinical Studies, Canterbury Christ Church University and Dr Shirley Bach, Head of the School of Nursing and Midwifery at the University of Brighton

Clinical Judgement and Decision Making in Nursing	ISBN 978 1 84445 468 6
Critical Thinking and Writing for Nursing Students	ISBN 978 1 84445 366 5
Evidence-based Practice in Nursing	ISBN 978 1 84445 369 6
Information Skills for Nursing Students	ISBN 978 1 84445 381 8
Reflective Practice in Nursing	ISBN 978 1 84445 371 9
Succeeding in Research Project Plans and Literature Reviews for Nursing Students	ISBN 978 0 85725 264 7
Successful Professional Portfolios for Nursing Students	ISBN 978 0 85725 457 3
Understanding Research for Nursing Students	ISBN 978 1 84445 368 9

To order, contact our distributor: BEBC Distribution, Albion Close, Parkstone, Poole, BH12 3LL. Telephone: 0845 230 9000, email: learningmatters@bebc.co.uk. You can also find more information on each of these titles and our other learning resources at www.learningmatters. co.uk. Many of these titles are also available in various e-book formats, please visit our website for more information.

Leadership, Management and Team Working in Nursing

Shirley Bach
Peter Ellis

Learning Matters

First published in 2011 by Learning Matters Ltd

British Library Cataloguing in Publication Data
A CIP record for this book is available from the British Library

ISBN: 978 0 85725 453 5

This book is also available in the following ebook formats:

Adobe ebook ISBN: 978 0 85725 455 9
ePub ebook ISBN: 978 0 85725 454 2
Kindle ISBN: 978 0 85725 456 6

Cover and text design by Toucan Design
Project management and typesetting by 4word Ltd, Page & Print Production
Printed and bound in Great Britain by Short Run Press, Exeter, Devon

Learning Matters Ltd
20 Cathedral Yard
Exeter EX1 1HB
Tel: 01392 215560
E-mail: info@learningmatters.co.uk
www.learningmatters.co.uk

Contents

About the authors   *vi*

Introduction   1

1   Experience of management and leadership   5

2   Teams and team work   20

3   Working with individuals in teams   37

4   Conflict management and negotiation skills   55

5   Coaching, mentoring and clinical supervision   72

6   Frameworks for management and leadership   88

7   Improving care, change management and entrepreneurial skills   105

8   Creating a learning environment   124

9   Developing confidence as a manager and leader   136

Glossary   151

References   153

Index   158

About the authors

Dr Shirley Bach is Head of the School of Nursing and Midwifery at the University of Brighton. Previously she was head of postgraduate studies and has developed curricula for undergraduate and pre-registration courses in a variety of subject domains. Nursing experience outside of the UK, in acute care settings and in primary care, has given her a rich background from which to draw in supporting the curricula of future nursing courses. In the past, she has specialised in health psychology and the application of psychology to health and illness settings. Recently, she has developed an interest in new learning technologies.

Shirley has 14 years experience as a manager and teaches leadership and management on pre and post qualifying nursing courses. She has written another book in the *Transforming Nursing Practice series – Communication and Interpersonal Skills in Nursing*, 2nd edition (with Alec Grant).

Peter Ellis is Senior Lecturer in Adult Nursing at Canterbury Christ Church University where he teaches leadership and management, research and other subjects at pre-registration, post-registration and postgraduate level. Prior to joining Canterbury, Peter was Senior Nurse – Renal Outpatients and Research Projects Manager at King's College Hospital, London. He has written two other books in the *Transforming Nursing Practice* series – *Understanding Research for Nursing Students* and *Evidence Based Practice in Nursing*.

Introduction

This book introduces you to the concepts of leadership and management in nursing, explains why this topic is relevant for you, and links it to the NMC standards and essential skills clusters for pre-registration nursing.

Who should read this book?

This book is written for anyone working in health and social care who has some element of leadership and management in their role. Most specifically, the book is aimed at student nurses who are trying to make sense of the leadership and management which happens in the places where they work. New leaders and managers will find the book useful in providing a framework within which to structure their thinking about what they do and why.

What is it about?

This focus is on those attitudes, values and practices which serve to make for good leadership and management. Throughout the book, we as authors are concerned to challenge our readers to adopt an approach to leadership and management which centres on the human elements of the role. Readers are prompted to think about the ideals which brought them into nursing practice in the first place and consider how these might apply to what they do as potential and actual leaders or managers of people.

Why is it important?

Leadership is an integral feature of the work of every nurse. This applies to student nurses developing their leadership skills within the ward or clinic team as much as it does to the ward manager or matron. It is important to engage with and develop leadership skills early on in your nursing career as the dispositions, attitudes and skills of leadership do not suddenly appear overnight following promotion. Clearly the values student nurses bring to their training and their interactions with patients and clients are the same, perhaps better defined, values as those that apply to the effective and ethical management of fellow professionals.

How is it structured?

The format of the book reflects the way in which we see the need for students to think about what it means to be led, to work in a team and to lead and manage development. The individual chapters can be read and understood on their own merits, but read together they help form a coherent picture of what we believe good leadership and management practice looks like.

Chapter 1, *Experience of management and leadership*, highlights the importance of remembering and understanding what it means to be led and what this might mean for the way in which you subsequently choose to lead.

Chapter 2, *Teams and team work*, identifies what teams are, why they exist and how they can work better towards their common goals. The next chapter, *Working with individuals in teams*, introduces the roles and responsibilities of individuals within teams and issues such as recruitment and delegation. In Chapter 4, *Conflict management and negotiation skills*, the different personality types that may operate within teams are described, and ways of managing conflict in the team and other settings are explored.

Chapter 5, *Coaching, mentoring and clinical supervision*, investigates the role of the leader or manager in supporting team members. This is followed by a chapter on *Frameworks for management and leadership*, which identifies and examines some theories of leadership and management and their interconnectedness.

Chapter 7, *Improving care, change management and entrepreneurial skills* , presents theories which may underpin leadership practice in relationship to the instigation and management of change; while Chapter 8, *Creating a learning environment*, considers the value of understanding the culture within which teams work and the impact this may have on the successful working of the team.

In Chapter 9, *Developing confidence as a manager and leader*, some of the tasks and roles undertaken by the leader or manager are laid bare. The chapter goes on to look at how these might be used to develop certainty in what they do for the developing leader.

NMC Standards for Pre-registration Nursing Education and Essential Skills Clusters

The Nursing and Midwifery Council (NMC) Standards of Competence provide guidance on the abilities and dispositions nursing students need to develop in order to meet the requirements for registration. As well as the Standards of Competence, the NMC identifies skills nursing students need to develop during their training; these Essential Skills Clusters (ESCs) are necessary for students to enter registered practice as capable practitioners.

This book identifies some of the competencies as essential, which relate to leadership and management and which student nurses need in order to attain NMC registration. These competencies and ESCs are presented at the start of each chapter so the reader can focus on how the content of each chapter contributes to their own competence and skill development. All of the competencies and ESCs in this book relate to the *generic standards* that all nursing students must achieve prior to registration. This book includes the latest taken from the *Standards for*

Pre-registration Nursing Education. Links to the relevant 2010 standards are outlined on the Learning Matters website page for this book, www.learningmatters.co.uk/nursing.

Activities

The activities contained within each chapter of the book form an integral part of the learning and development strategy for each chapter. Readers will get the most benefit from each chapter if they engage with the activities fully and in the order they are presented. The activities are designed to help illustrate the nature and reality of some of the theory presented and to bring to life some of the situations, scenarios and associated skills and competencies described. Some of the activities require readers to seek out new information and new experiences. Engagement with this process adds not only to the development of understanding but also potentially to confidence.

Reflection on the chapter content and on the activities contained within them is an important and integral part of the process of the student nurse's development as a leader of people. Some activities require readers to come to some decision or understanding for themselves, while others have some suggested answers presented at the end of the chapter. Readers are encouraged to consider each activity for themselves before reading the suggested answers in order that they come to some understanding of their own level of comprehension of the content of the chapter as well as their own personal and professional development.

Other features

The text also includes case studies and scenarios, research summaries and the necessary theory. There is also a glossary of terms at the end of the book. Glossary entries will be in bold blue type the first time they appear.

Acknowledgements

Peter Ellis wishes to pay tribute to his friend Stan – a true leader – and to thank his wife and children for giving him the space to write.

Chapter 1
Experience of management and leadership

NMC Standards for Pre-registration Nursing Education

This chapter will address the following competencies:

Domain 1: Professional values

2. All nurses must practise in a holistic, non-judgmental, caring and sensitive manner that avoids assumptions, supports social inclusion; recognises and respects individual choice; and acknowledges diversity. Where necessary, they must challenge inequality, discrimination and exclusion from access to care.

5. All nurses must fully understand the nurse's various roles, responsibilities and functions, and adapt their practice to meet the changing needs of people, groups, communities and populations.

Domain 4: Leadership, management and team working

4. All nurses must be self-aware and recognise how their own values, principles and assumptions may affect their practice. They must maintain their own personal and professional development, learning from experience, through supervision, feedback, reflection and evaluation.

Essential Skills Clusters

This chapter will address the following ESCs:

Cluster: Organisational aspects of care

12. People can trust the newly registered graduate nurse to respond to their feedback and a wide range of other sources to learn, develop and improve services.

14. People can trust the newly registered graduate nurse to be an autonomous and confident member of the multi-disciplinary or multi agency team and to inspire confidence in others.

Chapter aims

After reading this chapter, you will be able to:

* identify some of the values which underpin nurse leadership and management;

continued overleaf...

5

continued...

- understand how the experience of *being led* affects the ways in which we choose to lead and manage in nursing;
- comment on why leadership and management in nursing is important;
- begin to create a coherent picture of what leadership and management structures in nursing look like.

Introduction

The purpose of this chapter is to increase your awareness of the personal and professional values that influence the ways in which managers and leaders should behave. The chapter will both challenge and reinforce some of the assumptions you hold about the ways in which leaders and managers function.

Our **values** and assumptions about leadership and management are to a great extent derived from our experiences of leading and managing, and of being led and managed. This means they will reflect our personal interpretation of what happened during the process. It is important that, at the start of any quest to understand leadership and management, we should first understand ourselves and our motivations. Only in this way can we hope to understand the context of leadership and management and the behaviours and motivations of those we seek to lead.

As well as exploring the context of values in relation to leadership and management, this chapter will also explore some of the characteristics of leaders and managers. These descriptions will reflect the characteristics leadership and management theorists believe good managers and leaders should portray, including their personality traits. After examining these characteristics, you will be encouraged to formulate a picture of how you believe a good leader or manager should behave, and the essential qualities you believe they should exhibit within the nursing context.

(For more detailed discussion of theories and frameworks for leadership and management, and how they can be adopted and adapted by you to help meet the challenges of nurse leadership in the twenty-first century, see Chapter 6.)

A further important theme of this chapter is why leadership and management are important in nursing practice now and in the future, as well as how an understanding of them can contribute to your personal and professional development.

Towards the end of the chapter, some of the reasons for the existence of different leadership and management roles in nursing are introduced and discussed. You are invited to collect some data on the nursing structures where you work and how these impact on the work you and your colleagues do.

Understanding context and values

Our ideas and opinions about good leadership and management are coloured to a great extent by our personal experiences of leadership and management, whether we are managers, leaders or team members. The assumptions we draw about management and leadership styles and behaviours are also affected by our understanding of what is going on and the motivations behind the management and leadership styles we adopt or see adopted. The inability to understand why a certain approach to management or leadership has been adopted can lead to misconceptions and misunderstandings; this is something an understanding of the context of nurse leadership and management allows us to see beyond. Sometimes this context is better developed as we gain more experience as nurses and reflect thoughtfully on what these experiences actually mean.

Activity 1.1 *Reflection*

When you first came into nursing and went into practice for the first time, how did you feel about the efforts made by the staff to get frail, elderly patients to engage in self care? For example, encouraging elderly patients to get out of bed in the morning and to get washed and dressed. Now you understand a bit more about the purpose and nature of nursing, have you changed your view? Why?

There are some possible answers and thoughts at the end of the chapter.

Understanding why something is done in a particular way in a given situation allows us to understand the context of an action in the clinical setting. As shown in Activity 1.1, a developing understanding of the nature of nursing and what it means to nurse helps us to make sense of the world of work and the roles in which we find ourselves. The same is true of leadership and management where actions taken out of context may appear to be wrong.

One of the enduring difficulties for student nurses can be to understand the provision of care beyond the individual. Often the context of nursing management and leadership is about achieving the best outcomes on a regular, recurring and equitable basis for the many. The need to achieve good outcomes for the many rather than the few may help us to understand the context of a management or leadership style we see before us. This view is one which can only develop if we are willing and able to question the leadership and management practices we see around us and are then willing and able to reflect on the answers we find.

Case study: The newly qualified nurse

Julius is a newly qualified staff nurse working on a busy cardiology ward. Julius is irritated by the apparent inactivity of the ward sister Deirdre, who spends vast amounts of time in the office doing what to him appears to be endless and pointless paperwork instead of providing patient care. Julius confronts Deirdre about the lack of time she spends on the ward and suggests much of the time she is doing nothing of value while she is 'hiding away' in her office.

continued overleaf...

---

continued...

Deirdre understands the point Julius is making and is wise enough to appreciate that his frustrations arise not out of malice towards her but as a result of his inexperience and lack of understanding of what it takes to keep a busy ward functioning smoothly. Deirdre takes Julius into her office and shows him some of the tasks she has to perform on a regular basis which include: writing the duty roster, completing staff appraisals, entering patient dependency scores on to a monitoring database, ordering stock and overseeing staff development planning.

Deirdre explains to Julius she too is frustrated by the lack of time she has to provide care on a daily basis: that, she explains, is after all why she came into nursing. But she also understands her role now is less about providing care and more about facilitating the delivery of care. Deirdre explains she achieves this through: supporting the staff on the ward to improve using appraisals and accessing appropriate education and development; rostering to allow for a good work-life balance and by managing the budget while ensuring the hospital administrators know what the needs of the ward are by recording the level of dependency of the patients and the stock requirements. She explains she sees her role as supporting the staff to care for the patients, and if she did not do the necessary tasks then there would be chaos.

Julius concedes he had not looked at things in this way and he needed to understand the wider context before criticising.

From this example we can see that leadership and management often involve the need to see the bigger picture – which may not always be evident to members of the team. In order to understand the challenges and benefits that accrue from good leadership, it is necessary to understand something of the context of nursing leadership and management.

Clearly from this example we can see that one of the necessary qualities of a good manager or leader is the ability to see the bigger picture and anticipate and plan what the team will be doing and how they will do it. Leadership and management is therefore as much a forward looking activity as it is about managing what is happening in the here and now. One of the characteristics of a good manager or leader is understanding what it is they want to achieve and being able to communicate this, and perhaps effectively delegate associated tasks, to the team.

What we should remember at this stage is one of the most important things that drives us as nurses to achieve the goals we do is our values. Before we explore some more about the context of nursing leadership and management, we should stop for a moment to reflect on these values we have as humans, nurses, leaders or managers and see what impact they might have on leadership and management in nursing.

Evidently, within the case study above, Deirdre had not forgotten the values that took her into nursing in the first place. What had changed then for Deirdre as she moved from a clinical role to a more managerial post was simply the way in which these values were allowed to express themselves. In order to continually develop as nurses, leaders and managers, it is important not only that we question our values from time to time, but that we are also able to express what these values are and refine them in discussion with our colleagues.

Activity 1.2   *Decision making*

Take some time to think about the values you have as a nurse. Now think about how these values show themselves in the ways in which you act when in the clinical setting. Next time you are in practice, ask your team leader or ward manager what values they hold and how they think they express them in practice. Now compare the lists looking for areas of overlap and areas of difference. What do you notice about the similarities and differences between your list of values and corresponding actions and the leader's values and actions?

There are some possible answers and thoughts at the end of the chapter.

What is clear about the values of practising nurses, ward managers and more senior nursing staff is they should, and to a great extent do, share similar values and goals. The role of the leader or manager should be to facilitate the team in the achievement of these goals. Evidently where there are differences in the values and goals of the team and the team leader then difficulties will arise. When nurses or nurse leaders forget what their values are, then they will lose sight of what it is they are trying to achieve.

Sometimes it is hard to know what exactly our values are or the limits to which they can be stretched. One method for understanding our values as potential leaders or managers is to ask ourselves hypothetical questions the answers to which can be searching and difficult for us. The answers to these difficult questions enable us however to understand what sort of person we are and what motivates us as humans, nurses and managers. Understanding our own values and underlying motivations will then tell us something about what is likely to motivate and guide the actions of those that we may be called upon to lead.

Activity 1.3   *Reflection*

Imagine you are working in a nursing home on nights. You are tired, having already worked six shifts in a row. One of the residents, Jane, who is in her late 80s, has been in the home for some time as a result of having had a stroke. Jane needs to be turned two hourly to avoid her developing pressure sores, but you and the nurse you are working with decide to turn her just occasionally. You justify this to yourselves by saying this avoids disturbing her sleep and it also protects your backs. At the end of the shift you turn her and record in her notes that you have done so two hourly throughout the night. She has not developed a pressure sore so what is the harm?

Now consider this: you turn her at the end of the night and discover that a small area has broken down on her left hip. Is this your fault? If the matron asks if you have turned her two hourly as stated in the care plan, what will you say? You could say you turned her two hourly – this would not change anything for Jane, but would make your life easier.

Alternatively you go to turn her at the end of the night shift only to discover that she has died some time during the night. She has been dead for a while judging from how cold she is and that blood is pooling on the side she was lying on. You know you can just claim that

continued overleaf...

continued...

you found her earlier in the night and prepare her body quickly before the day staff come in to work. Surely this will not change anything; no one will be hurt, will they?

Which, if any, of these scenarios are acceptable? Does the blame attached to any of them change because of the outcome? What does your choice of actions say about you? What values are being displayed here? How do they compare with the values you expressed in Activity 1.2?

There are some possible answers and thoughts at the end of the chapter.

Examining examples such as this enable us to see the bigger picture. They are also helpful for us in developing an increasing awareness of our own values as they relate to being led and managed and then conversely to us leading or managing. In part our values will be mirrored in the sort of person we are and how we see the world in general, but they will also shape the way in which the world sees us. Of course it might be equally bad if a nurse were to follow policy and procedure blindly with no thought about the consequences. In this scenario, as in many leadership and management situations, deviating from what we know to be right (i.e. ignoring our values) can have dire consequences for those we care for.

Activity 1.4   *Leadership and management*

You are working on a medical admissions unit and have asked a colleague, Emma, to go round and do the observations. She takes the temperature, pulse and blood pressure of every patient on the unit as asked. About an hour later you ask if all the observations were OK. Emma replies that the lady in the first bed had a temperature of 39°C. You ask why she had not informed you of this immediately. She replies that it was her job to do all of the observations as you asked, and that is what she has done.

What does this scenario tell you about managing and leading people in the clinical setting? What does this tell you about the need to understand what we do and why? Is there a place for understanding values of care in this scenario?

There are some possible answers and thoughts at the end of the chapter.

By now you should have developed a fairly clear picture of the values that you believe underpin what you do as a student nurse. You may well also have some insight into the values of those around you and the impact that working among other nurses has on the development of your own value set. What it is important to understand is that for a leader or manager to be effective there is a requirement for there to be some degree of overlap between their values and the values of their team, and the team must be aware of this.

It is probably fair to say that in order to become an effective leader or manager of people, we first must know ourselves as well as having some insight into how others see us. Part of leadership or management is presentation of self to others and encouraging others to follow our lead by behaving in ways and displaying values that others admire and can identify with – creating a situation where others wish to follow. When you think about it a leader without followers is just a person working alone!

How we see ourselves and others see us

To understand how we see ourselves and how this compares to how others see us it is worth looking at the work of Joseph Luft and Harry Ingham, whose 'Johari window' illustrates the point about what we know about ourselves and what others know about us.

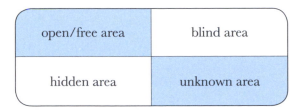

Figure 1.1: The Johari window
Source: Adapted from Luft and Ingham (1955) page 10.

What the Johari window allows us to see is how much of the perceptions and knowledge we have about ourselves is also seen and shared by others:

- the open/free area refers to what we know about ourselves and what is also known by other people – it is our public face;
- the blind area is the area of our personality we are blind to but which others can see – our blind spot;
- the hidden area is what we know about ourselves but what we keep hidden from others, sometimes called the 'avoided self' or 'facade';
- the unknown area refers to what is unknown to both ourself and to others (which can be regarded as an area for potential development and self exploration).

What is interesting about this model is it shows us there is great potential for us as individuals to lack understanding of ourselves as much as there is potential for other people not to understand us. To some extent we can manage the view others have of us as individuals by allowing them to see what we want them to see and by managing our behaviours at work and in our private lives. On the other hand, people are often aware of issues with our values and personality that we sometimes are aware of and sometimes not.

Being able to adapt who we are and how we behave at work is part of the process of socialising to be both a nurse and a member of society at large. By being aware of our values and acting upon them we allow ourselves the ability to become someone we want to become and potentially to develop the traits that will help us to develop as a person, a nurse and over time as a manager or leader.

Activity 1.5   *Communication*

In order to get some idea of how your view of yourself is similar to, or differs from, that of other people, undertake the following exercise which may tell you something about how you communicate with and are perceived by other people: Choose five words to describe what sort of person you believe yourself to be and write these down. Ask a number of

continued overleaf...

continued...

people who you know to choose five words which describe what sort of person you are and write these down. Include fellow students, lecturers, mentors and other people you work with. Examine the lists for similarities and differences and assign the responses to the various boxes of the Johari window and consider what this says about how your perception of self concurs or contrasts with the views of others.

Since this is based on your own thoughts and reflections, there is no specimen answer at the end of the chapter.

Activity 1.5 will help you to see that sometimes people see good and sometimes bad things about us which we may or may not see for ourselves. The lesson for the would-be leader is to learn to change the negatives that we can change and to manage the areas of our personality that we cannot. You should also be prepared to take on board positive insights and use these to continue to improve your relationships with others.

What are the characteristics of a good leader or manager?

What makes a good leader/manager has been explored by many theorists and academics over the years. Some of the early theorists identified characteristics such as physical size, strength and 'presence' (Wright, 1996). Other characteristics and traits that have been favoured include intelligence, personality type such as extroversion and charisma and other interpersonal skills.

Certainly it is true that being charismatic and intelligent help with the processing of ideas and in communication with others can help a leader. But as we have seen above there must be more to being a good nurse, good leader or good manager than these superficial qualities alone. Sometimes extreme examples allow us to see things that are perhaps not clear to us in the day-to-day process of being managed or led.

Activity 1.6   *Reflection*

Reflect on some of the well known and successful leaders you know from history, perhaps Winston Churchill, Nelson Mandela, Martin Luther King or Florence Nightingale. What characteristics do they share that makes them great leaders? Why are they thought of as great individuals as well as successful leaders?

Next think about some of the other successful leaders from history like Adolf Hitler, Napoleon Bonaparte, Joseph Stalin or Saddam Hussein. What characteristics made them successful leaders? Why are they thought of as immoral leaders?

There are some possible answers and thoughts at the end of the chapter.

Interestingly from the examples of good leaders given above, none of them were particularly impressive physically, so their ability to lead and inspire has to be explained in some other way. Certainly this observation calls into question some of the early physical appearance theories of what makes a good leader. Clearly there may be issues relating to their charisma and intellect that attracted other people to them.

What we can see about the leaders in activity 1.6, and what perhaps others know about some of them that they do not see for themselves, is the leaders we admire have a vision of something better for the people they lead. In the case of Mandela and Luther King this was freedom from oppression and the achievement of equality of status and human rights. The pursuit of these values and the veracity with which they pursued them gives us a clue as to one other quality we might admire in a leader: **integrity** (Frankel, 2008). In this sense integrity may be understood as acting in a manner that reflects the values, ethics and morals that an individual believes to be important.

Integrity alone is not enough however. Hitler, Stalin and Saddam all perhaps believed in what they were doing; in that sense they had integrity. What is interesting about what they believed and what they set out to achieve was that it was often more about achieving power for themselves than it was about achieving what was right or something that benefits others.

What is missing therefore is an understanding about what this integrity and leadership should be aimed at achieving. Leaders and managers are the figureheads of teams and teams exist to get a job done (Ward, 2003). In nursing this job is about providing care for others in a manner that reflects the positive values we hold as humans and as nurses. For a nurse leader or manager, therefore, integrity of action means leading and managing in a manner that reflects the values of care which are part of what being a nurse is about and which you have identified for yourself in Activity 1.2.

Activity 1.7   *Reflection*

It is perhaps worth reflecting on the answers you gave to Activity 1.2 and comparing them to what you have learnt so far in this chapter. You should be able to see some commonalities between the ideas and therefore have some ideas of what being a good nurse leader or manager is all about.

Since this is based on your own observations there is no specimen answer at the end of the chapter.

So far in this chapter we have seen that being a good leader or manager in nursing is about the expression of the same values of care that being a good nurse require. What changes when one moves from being a nurse to a nurse leader or manager is the way in which these values are expressed through what we do and how we behave towards others. The consistency of the values between nursing and nurse leadership/management demonstrate integrity. It is perhaps a sad fact that those nurse leaders and managers who we see losing sight of their values are the ones we least admire. The report into the failings at the Mid Staffordshire Hospitals identified poor leadership coupled with clinical staff: 'accepting standards of care…that should not have been tolerated' (Clews, 2010). The collective failing here was that clinically trained managers did not support their staff as well as they might and the managers and leaders, as well as their staff, allowed the standards of care to slip below a level reflective of the true values of nursing.

One of the challenges of this book is for you to recognise and acknowledge the values that you have as a nursing student and to think about how you will continue to exercise these values throughout your nursing career.

Structures of nurse leadership

What we have not discussed so far are the structures that relate to the exercise of leadership and management. Clearly a manager occupies a formal role. The role of the manager is conferred upon the individual by an organisation and its staff are responsible to the manager by virtue of their contract of employment with the organisation – often called **legitimate power** (first identified by French and Raven in 1960). How these lines of responsibility are created and what they mean in practice should be clearer after the next activity.

Activity 1.8   *Research*

To understand the lines of responsibility that form part of a contract look at the programme handbook for the programme you are on. There will be clear guidelines about some things you can and cannot do as a university student. There will be identified individuals to whom you would have to answer should you break these rules. This forms part of your contract with the university and ultimately with the Nursing and Midwifery Council (NMC) in relation to the fitness to practice criteria.

Alternatively, if you have a contract of employment you may notice it identifies the person to whom you are answerable, usually a line manager.

As this is based on your own observations there is no specimen answer at the end of the chapter.

Managerial power and responsibility, as you can see from having done Activity 1.8, are therefore formalised within the contract of employment or training. They are validated by the fact that we choose to submit to these contracts of our own free will, usually because they will confer some benefit on us (in the case of a job through being paid and in the case of being a student nurse in gaining a qualification). Similarly, as nurses we agree to be bound by our code of conduct and other regulations pertaining to nursing (NMC, 2008).

Within most organisations there are a number of managers at different levels who have different responsibilities for different organisational activities. These managers report to a more senior manager who in turn reports to more senior management. Such structures are formalised and are usually created in order to allow for the overseeing of the functions of the organisation. Each tier within the system of management should be aware of their responsibilities and the limits of their powers in fulfilling the tasks associated with these roles. It is often helpful for the novice nurse to have some idea of what the structure of the organisation they work in looks like.

In Chapter 8 we discuss a little about cultures of care and you may find it useful to look up Charles Handy's work on cultures in order to inform your thinking about the formal and informal management structures which can exist in health and social care.

Activity 1.9   *Evidence-based practice and research*

Try to find out something about the management structure in the hospital in which you are placed. There may be a diagram that shows the relative management positions

continued opposite...

---

continued...

(sometimes called an organogram); then try to find out what the main responsibilities are of the people in the various roles you have identified. You might also like to do something similar for a ward or other practice area you work in so you can get an overview of who is responsible for what.

As this is based on your own observation there is no specimen answer at the end of the chapter.

So we can see being a manager is a formalised position that is conferred by position within an organisation. Being a leader on the other hand may or may not be the result of position within a team or organisation. How can this be?

As we will see elsewhere in the book, leadership is in many instances one of the roles of a manager; think about the ward managers in the areas you have worked who as well as managing the ward also lead the team. Think also about the areas where you have worked where individuals who occupy a junior role in a team exercise leadership. Sometimes then the leadership function is one of the roles of the manager, while on other occasions something else is at work.

How then do some non-managers function as leaders? Essentially there are three answers to this question. First, some leaders, such as team leaders at the ward level, are designated leaders because they are more experienced than the other staff or they hold a higher, non-management, grade. They exercise the power of leadership also through virtue of the formal position they hold and the delegation of certain duties from their line manager. In this respect the power they exercise comes from the person who has delegated it to them – this is sometimes referred to as legitimate power. Legitimate power, within society and organisations, arises out of the fact that people vote for their leaders (in the societal sense) or they enter into contracts of work whereby they agree to be subject to the power of others within an organisation. The leadership roles within such arrangement are therefore legitimised by virtue of the fact that they represent a choice on the part of the people who are led by these elected, or contractual, leaders.

Second, other leaders exercise leadership in relation to specific projects or responsibilities within the team. For example, in many clinical areas there are link nurses with responsibility for such things as diabetes care, wound management or infection control. Again their power to act as leaders is in part conferred by the position they are asked to play in the team and is delegated from the team manager. The other reason they are a leader in their particular area is because they have specialist knowledge of the practice, procedures and guidelines that relate to whatever it is they are responsible for. In this situation a good leader will share the information the team needs to know to get the job done, a bad leader will not! Clearly then one of the characteristics of a leader is information management and good communication.

Third, there are those people who lead by virtue of their character. These charismatic individuals are the sort of people others like and respond to. They are able to motivate others and to get the team to follow them by virtue of who they are. They have a compelling vision of what should be done and how and have a conviction and surety about them which encourages others to follow their lead (Mahoney, 2001). They may not be in positions of formal power, but perhaps they have knowledge or good communication skills that single them out as people others like to follow.

What we can see in this case study is that, even within an essentially quite hierarchical structure, leadership can be found at all levels of the team. In this example there is a real danger that Eileen will lose control of the unit and Karen might overstep her own competence, role and responsibilities. Clearly one of the issues that arises out of this scenario is accountability. Eileen as a registered nurse is accountable for what she does as well as the actions of her team, especially the untrained members. Karen as a care assistant is not accountable for her actions in the same way, but is responsible to her employer (actually Eileen) for what she does.

In this scenario the power which Karen exercises is not strictly speaking legitimate. As with all members of the team she has roles and responsibilities for which she may need to exercise the power given to her by virtue of her position. It may be that Karen has the power to order stores and perhaps organise transport, but these are subject to the need to recognise the roles and responsibilities of other members of the team who may need support in developing the skills necessary for them to operate effectively within their identified role.

It may be argued therefore that the leadership that Karen exercises is in this instance a bad thing. Karen is perhaps motivated to get the immediate job done, but perhaps misses some of the bigger picture issues, such as the quality of the dialysis, that she is not trained in and not in a position to understand. Because Karen takes over the day-to-day running of the unit, she is also both undermining Eileen and preventing her from developing into her new role. While in the short term this might appear to work, it is not a long-term solution.

Activity 1.10 *Reflection*

Take some time to think about the implications of this case study. What might this mean for the quality of nursing practice in the dialysis unit? What implications might this have for Eileen and for Karen in the long term? How are the other staff likely to feel about this situation?

There are some possible answers and thoughts at the end of the chapter.

So we have seen leadership and management within nursing can be broken down into many levels from the most senior member of the nursing team right through to the most junior and the qualities that make a good leader can be present at all levels. We have also seen that some managers fail to lead and that some leaders do not really have the formal position or power to do so.

Leading and managing: The policy context

Nursing is not undertaken in a vacuum. What we do as nurses and what nurse managers and leaders do occurs within a healthcare context and is subject to policy, procedure and guidelines. If leadership or management is about leading or managing a team to achieve certain outcomes, and within healthcare these outcomes are derived from policy and guidelines, then there is a need for nurse leaders and managers to not only be aware of what the guidelines are but also to act on them and ensure their team acts on them too.

Historically the caring professions had a great deal of autonomy over the ways in which they worked. In the past they set the standards by which their work was to be measured and audited and decided on clinical and non-clinical priorities. More recently, most notably following the policies of the Thatcher government and subsequently New Labour, clinical priority setting and the standards for care have been determined more centrally through government policy via agencies such as the National Institute for Health and Clinical Excellence (NICE) or via nationally drawn up structures for care such as the National Service Frameworks (NSFs). So part of the role of nurse leaders or managers will be having the ability to lead or manage their team through the change process to achieve the outcomes of care determined from outside of the team (see also Chapter 8).

As well as general policy and guidelines in the area of health, as nurses we are subject to policy and guidance from our professional body, the Nursing and Midwifery Council (NMC). In order to understand the context of leadership and management in nursing from the point of view of the NMC, it is worth familiarising yourself with the standards of proficiency and essential skills clusters identified at the start of each chapter and asking yourself how these apply within the context of each chapter. You may also wish to look at and reflect on how these ideas reflect the issues identified within other NMC documentation including the code of conduct (2008). Most especially this chapter has highlighted the need for nurse leaders to 'be self-aware and recognise how their own values, principles and assumptions may affect their practice' (NMC, 2010) as expressed in Competency 4 of the 'Leadership, management and team working' domain of the competency framework identified at the start of this chapter.

For example, in this chapter we have discussed some of the values that underpin nursing practice as well as leadership and management characteristics of the nurse leader/manager which may contribute to our development as good leaders and managers. These characteristics translate well from both the code of professional conduct and the standards of proficiency identified at the start of the chapter. What they validate is perhaps the most important message of the chapter: in order to become a good leader or manager of nurses it is important to remain grounded in the values, beliefs and behaviours that guide professional nursing practice.

> ### Chapter summary
>
> Rather than launch straight into a discussion about the nature of leadership and management in nursing, this chapter has sought to identify some of the values, beliefs and behaviours that might be associated with becoming a good nurse leader or manager. These characteristics have been compared and contrasted with some of the values which underpin being a good nurse. There is an explicit challenge within this chapter for you, to identify and confront the values you have as a nurse, a nursing student, a team member and a leader.
>
> An understanding of the context of care and of ourselves is an important first step on the road to becoming a competent leader of nurses; failure to understand what motivates us as individuals lays us open to external criticism. Furthermore, some of the skills and values we develop as nurses in clinical practice will translate well into leadership and management roles. It is never too soon for a student nurse to think about what type of leader/manager they want to be and to look around them for suitable role models to guide their development.

Activities: Brief outline answers

Activity 1.1 (page 7)

This reflection is not about understanding the rehabilitation of the elderly as such, it is about understanding context. As a new nurse you may consider asking people to undertake their own care as lazy nursing, because you consider nursing as a caring profession that does things for people. As you understand the nature of care better, you will see the same scenario in a different light, or context, as you understand that encouraging self care is about helping people address their care deficits and achieve the activities of daily living for themselves.

Activity 1.2 (page 9)

What you will notice is that the basic values of caring, moral behaviour, putting others before self, protection of rights, autonomy and dignity, etc. are common to both lists. What will be different is that the leader will attempt to achieve these aims through the way in which they lead. This will include acting as a role model and promoting the welfare of the team who in turn are expected to support these values one-to-one with patients and clients (Bondas, 2006). If you are still struggling to think about what your values are try some of the words above or choose some from this list: accountability, accuracy, calm, committed, decisive, fair, honesty, integrity, justice, open, reliable, team worker or truthfulness.

Activity 1.3 (page 9)

We hope you found none of these scenarios acceptable. On each occasion, regardless of the outcome, the choice being made was to avoid your duty to Jane to protect her from potential further physical harm. The values displayed here are self and not other regarding and are against everything that is to be found in the nursing code of conduct. At best, the scenario demonstrates lies being told and at worst a dereliction of the duty of care leading to harm to the patient. Some people might argue that as no harm ensued the first scenario might be alright, but the consequences that *could* accrue (as seen in the changes made to the scenario) show this to be wrong, regardless of any arguments about duty and outcomes.

Activity 1.4 (page 10)

This scenario suggests that as a manager or leader it is important not only to have team members who do what they are asked, but that they understand the purpose of what they are doing. There is a clear need here for the nurse to understand that doing observations is not enough in itself, it is acting on what is found that is important. The values which should drive the undertaking of such tasks is person centred care which requires that nurses not only undertake a task, but that they think about what that means for the patient or client.

Activity 1.6 (page 12)

Clearly one of the characteristics of good leaders is that people want to follow them. In many of the cases mentioned as potential positive role models, people choose to follow the leader because they believe in what they are doing. This is also the case for some of the examples of negative leadership role models given, so what is the difference? Some people would not choose to follow the likes of Hitler or Hussein, and although many did many more were coerced and forced to do so. Other people follow bad leaders because they generate a sense of belonging and solidarity perhaps at a time when there is uncertainty in the world. The integrity and ethicality of the examples of bad leaders is questionable at best and evil at worst. So perhaps integrity and morality are two of the things that we admire in good leaders?

Activity 1.10 (page 16)

While Karen does a good day-to-day job in making the dialysis unit function, there may be longer-term considerations to take into account. As we saw earlier in the chapter, one of the roles of a leader is operating within the bigger picture. This also resonates with the role of the trained nurse who not only has to account for the day-to-day running of the dialysis unit but also for the long-term health of the patients. So while it may be alright for the leader to allow someone else to take charge of some of the activities of the team, it is better if they are selective about who takes over what tasks and what they do. The staff in a scenario where it is uncertain who the real leader is will be confused, and may even be a little angry as they see someone without genuine authority taking control.

Further reading

Aldgate, J and Dimmock, B (2003) Managing to Care, in **Henderson, J and Atkinson, D** (eds) *Managing Care in Context*. London: Routledge.
This chapter explores the values of care as well as social inclusion.

Scott, J, Gill, A and Crowhurst, K (2008) *Effective Management in Long-term Care Organisations*. Exeter: Reflect Press.
See especially Chapter 4 on Leadership.

Useful websites

www.nursingleadership.org.uk/index.php
A good collection of leadership literature and developmental resources.

www.businessballs.com
An interesting and quirky leadership and management resources website.

www.kingsfund.org.uk/topics/leadership_and_management/index.html
Perhaps the leading UK healthcare think tank.

Chapter 2
Teams and team work

NMC Standards for Pre-registration Nursing Education

This chapter will address the following competencies:

Domain 4: Leadership, management and team working

6. All nurses must work independently as well as in teams. They must be able to take the lead in coordinating, delegating and supervising care safely, managing risk and remaining accountable for the care given.

7. All nurses must work effectively across professional and agency boundaries, actively involving and respecting others' contributions to integrate person-centred care. They must know when and how to communicate with and refer to other professionals and agencies in order to respect the choices of service users and others, promoting shared decision making, to deliver positive outcomes and to co-ordinate smooth, effective transition within and between services and agencies.

Essential Skills Clusters

This chapter will address the following ESCs:

Cluster: Organisational aspects of care

12. People can trust the newly registered graduate nurse to respond to their feedback and a wide range of other sources to learn, develop and improve services.

13. People can trust the newly registered graduate nurse to promote continuity when their care is to be transferred to another service or person.

15. People can trust the newly registered graduate nurse to safely delegate to others and to respond appropriately when a task is delegated to them.

16. People can trust the newly registered graduate nurse to safely lead, co-ordinate and manage care.

19. People can trust the newly registered graduate nurse to work to prevent and resolve conflict and maintain a safe environment.

Chapter aims

After reading this chapter, you will be able to:

- understand group roles and dynamics that impact team working and decision making;
- explore methods to evaluate effective team working;

continued opposite...

continued...

- consider the skills needed to lead teams, meetings and working groups;
- explore the role of interagency and interdisciplinary team working in healthcare delivery.

Introduction

In this chapter we will begin by looking at your experiences of working in a team and progress to how you will develop skills to manage and lead a team. Nurses are educated to make autonomous and independent professional decisions to manage patient care. At the same time, in healthcare environments, there will be an expectation for nurses to:

- work within teams of similar professionals (e.g. in wards or units);
- work with interdisciplinary teams (e.g. specialist teams, stroke management);
- manage and direct teams with specific tasks to be achieved (e.g. infection control);
- lead teams to introduce new ways of working or maintain high standards of care (e.g. implement initiatives to ensure care is dignified).

The chapter will examine how teams work and how to evaluate the effectiveness of teams working together. The different roles that team members assume in teams are covered next and skills for dealing with improving team working, difficulties with team members and communication are explored. In this section we also explore some of the theoretical positions that have helped to explain team members' behaviour based upon social psychology. The practicalities of leading team meetings are described and finally the role of interdisciplinary team working is discussed.

How teams work

Understanding group dynamics is the starting point to recognise how to work best within and with teams. Group dynamics is the study of how people come together and then work together in teams or groups to share a common goal and purpose. It may seem that some groups can work well together as if by magic, but it often needs a deeper understanding of the nature of groups and the individuals within them to ensure they work together.

Activity 2.1 *Reflection*

Think of the last team or group in which you worked with others. Think about what went on in that team or group and jot down those activities. Would you describe the experience as one where individuals came together for personally focused but unifying relationships, such as found in families, religious groups, political affiliations or students studying the same module? Or did the experience involve a number of persons associated together in specific work, activity or task?

continued overleaf...

continued...

If it was the former, this would be described as a group activity. If it was the latter, it would be described as a team. A team has:

- defined objectives;
- positive relationships operating in a supportive environment;
- a spirit of co-operation and collaboration that is focused on accomplishing something specific;
- specific outcomes that require the members to be effective.

There is no right or wrong answer to this activity. The aim is to help you differentiate between a team and a group.

In summary, a team is a number of people organised to function co-operatively as a group. By contrast, a group is deemed to be a number of people sharing something in common such as an interest, belief or political aim.

Activity 2.2   *Critical thinking*

Think about a time when you were involved in working in a team. This could be the experience you thought of in Activity 2.1 if it fits the definition of a team. Write down the main aim or purpose of the team. Think about whether or not the overall outcome was successful. Try to isolate the actions of the team leader and members that either helped to achieve or inhibited a successful outcome. Then make two lists: one for effective and one for ineffective activities. Divide the activities under each appropriate heading, then compare the two lists.

Try to isolate activities undertaken by individuals that helped the team's success. Then think about the activities that hindered the team working and think about what could have improved the hindering contributions. Do the same for the actions of the leader. Finally, consider your own contribution to the effectiveness of the team and consider whether you would improve on your performance as a result of standing back from the experience and analysing the parts that have been played in the team. Think particularly about the activities that made the team a success, and whether you would change your responses to be similar to these.

There is no right or wrong answer to this activity. The aim is to help you utilise a process of analysis to identify the various roles that play a part in effective team working. The next section discusses in more detail team effectiveness which will help you develop your team working skills.

Team effectiveness

When a team works well together there is a conspicuous difference in the work atmosphere. This is noticeable in several different ways, for example when team members:

- have a shared understanding of team goals and tasks;

- are willing to listen to each other;
- feel comfortable discussing their work with each other;
- handle disagreements positively and openly;
- give and receive feedback with respect for each others' feelings.

In contrast, an ineffective team can be dominated by a few members with strong views and opinions. This can mean other members feel isolated from the main purpose of the team, which in turn can lead to feelings such as disenfranchisement, boredom, a lack of engagement and commitment.

An overuse of rules and regulations can lead to a stifling of informal relationship building, a process that is necessary to achieve team harmony and a supportive atmosphere. For example, each team will have a set of norms to guide it on how each person should be addressed – whether by organisational title and family name, or by first name. Another example might occur when a team has devised a specific method of dealing with patients' personal effects that fits fundamentally with the principles of the organisation's policy but which have been tested and proven to be less than practical given the nature of the unit – such as an emergency care unit where people are being constantly moved around. On the other hand, a leader needs to know which institutional or legal regulations have to be followed for procedures and patient safety to be maintained. Individual team members should also be aware of their own professional responsibilities, guided by professional codes of conduct such as the Nursing and Midwifery Council (NMC) code for nurses and midwives. Acknowledging individuals' responsibility also reinforces a sense of professional autonomy that can contribute positively to (or indeed detract from) team working.

Conflicts and disagreements are uncomfortable situations to deal with in a team. However, if not dealt with these situations can lead to team members avoiding each other and suppressing negative feelings. This, in turn, can lead to resentment and frustration. So it is important to look at disagreements as opportunities for improving team relationships: by talking through differences and discussing alternative ways of working together. Team leaders can facilitate these discussions or they can be between the individuals provided ground rules are established and resolution of the differences is made a focal objective. A helpful team activity for dealing with differences is for the team to develop a team code of co-operation. (See useful websites section at the end of this chapter, also Chapter 4, for further information on dealing with conflict.)

Giving feedback on performance to team members (whether you are a leader or from one co-worker to another) is an activity that, for an effective team, needs to be integrated into discussions about work. Effective feedback can enhance performance and improve the outcomes for the team. But it can so easily seem like negative criticism. This is especially so when it may be about the work of a superior, a more experienced colleague or towards a less experienced colleague who is developing their confidence in participating in the team. Chapter 3 looks more closely at working with individuals within teams, and Chapter 5 at issues around coaching and mentoring colleagues.

Negative or destructive criticism that is personal and hurtful has the potential to erupt and create discordant relationships that in turn lead to resentment and hidden feelings. One way for a team to learn to work with constructive feedback is to practise, or role play, in a simulated situation by giving feedback to one another to experience what it feels like; and to generate or become accustomed to phrases that are acceptable to convey feedback to one another in a respectful manner, as shown in Table 2.1 below.

Characteristic	Effective	Ineffective
Leadership	Has a clear idea of what the team needs to do to achieve its goals, facilitates team working in a supportive atmosphere	Unclear idea of direction, does not allow team members to express ideas, does not capitalise on individual strengths in the team, overly autocratic
Environment	Informal, open	Indifferent, tense, strained
Discussion	Shared, focused on getting the job done and making improvements, actively listening to each other	Unfocused, dominated by a few strong characters, no active listening
Response to points of view	Respectful, encouraging, trusting each other's judgement	Patronising and judgemental, over critical, mistrustful
Decision making	Reached by consensus, general agreement acceptable, dissenters tolerated, diverse views accepted	Lack of consensus and discussion, lack of flexibility or appreciation of differing perceptions, reliance on only majority acceptance as basis for agreement
Feedback	Constructive, honest, directed towards problem solving	Personal, destructive, aimed at creating embarrassment
Tasks, responsibilities	Clear, agreed by all despite some disagreement	Unclear, resented by dissenting members
Feelings	Open for discussion, exploration and support	Hidden, potentially explosive

Table 2.1: Summary of effective and ineffective team characteristics

Source: Adapted from Yoder-Wise, P (2007) Elsevier, page 345.

Activity 2.3   *Reflection*

Reflecting back on Activity 2.2 and your own list of effective and ineffective behaviours, compare your analysis with the summary above and see if you can add to the summary or use the summary to reflect further on the activities of the team you were analysing.

This activity relates to your own experience and reflections, so there is no right or wrong answer and no outline answer at the end of the chapter.

Team dynamics and processes

The manner in which team members engage with each other and the factors that affect the team functioning well together are crucial aspects of effective team working. It is customary for there to be a designated team leader who will guide the team's performance and set the tone for how a team will work together. There are occasions, however, when a team will be self directed and led jointly by members who have similar status or responsibilities, such as in a multi-disciplinary group.

Norms

Most teams develop norms, which are the informal rules of behaviour shared and enforced by team members. These norms are developed by the teams as a form of self regulation to enable stable team functioning and survival. Norms are often linked to expected contributions from individual performances. For example, a student nurse's contribution to the team will be bounded by supernumerary or experience of the course. A healthcare assistant will have expectations of the role of a qualified nurse and will support the qualified nurse with agreed activities or parameters.

However, these parameters may vary from unit to unit and ward to ward, depending on the nature of the work or the experience of the team members. Understanding these different parameters can sometimes lead to misunderstandings because of the variations and student nurses or new team members will need to find out the norms of any group by discussion and reference to unit protocols. Examples of other norms may be about when breaks are taken, how shifts are negotiated, how to prevent embarrassment by being loyal to the team, and how collectively held values or principles are best expressed.

Roles

A role is an expected set of behaviours that is characteristic of a specific function in the team. Individuals may have an inherent tendency to perform a role, such as a nurturing role; alternatively, roles may be informally ascribed by the group or formally designated by the leader. Sullivan and Decker (2009, page 152) suggest roles can be divided into either task roles or nurturing roles and they are set out in the two following tables.

Initiator-contributor	Redefines problems and offers solutions, clarifies objectives, suggests agenda items and maintains time limits
Information seeker	Pursues descriptive baseline information for the team's work
Information giver	Expands information given by sharing experiences and making inferences
Opinion seeker	Explores viewpoints that clarify or reflect the values of other members' suggestions

continued overleaf...

continued...

Opinion giver	Conveys to group members what their essential values should be
Elaborator	Predicts outcomes and provides illustrations or expands suggestions, clarifying how they could work
Co-ordinator	Links ideas or suggestions offered by others
Orienter	Summarises the group's discussions and actions
Evaluator critic	Appraises the quantity and quality of the team's accomplishments against set standards
Energiser	Motivates the group to accomplish, qualitatively and quantitatively, the team's goals
Procedural technician	Supports team activity by arranging the environment and providing necessary equipment
Recorder	Documents the team's progress, actions and achievements

Table 2.2: Task roles

Encourager	Compliments members for their opinions and contributions to the team
Harmoniser	Relieves tensions and conflicts
Compromiser	Submits own position or views to maintain team harmony
Gate keeper	Stimulates discussion to enable all team members to communicate and participate, without allowing any one member to dominate
Group observer	Notices team processes and dynamics and informs the team of them
Follower	Passively attends meetings, listens to discussions and accepts the team's decisions

Table 2.3: Nurturing roles

Task roles keep the team focused on the objectives or functions of the team whereas nurturing roles are facilitative or concerned with maintaining interpersonal needs. Team members may adopt more than one role. A team leader may wish to accentuate one role in place of another to improve team functioning or alternatively to suppress a role that becomes over emphasised. This is where the team leader assumes the nature of a conductor of an orchestra to utilise the different talents of the team, possibly at different times, to achieve a successful performance.

Meredith Belbin (2010) continues to be one of the major contributors to team role theory. Based on research into dysfunctional teams in the 1970s, Belbin found that effective teams were founded upon individual behaviours. The research was developed to control team dynamics; however, the researchers found that the difference between success and failure was not based on intellect but on separate clusters of behaviour, each forming a specific contribution to effective team working.

They went on to identify nine team roles; each was essential to the team and necessary to create a balance of roles. In addition, it was discovered that each role had a flip side or weakness, which was not always productive but within the team this would be tolerated because of the strength that would go with it. (See the useful websites list at the end of the chapter for more information on Belbin's work.)

Influence of social systems on teams

Teams do not work in isolation. In healthcare they are often located in organisations or as subsets of other larger team structures such as departments or divisions. These background factors need to be taken into consideration for a full analysis of team dynamics (personal relationships) and processes (actions directed towards a specific aim). The sociologist George Homans (1961) used a systemic model to describe what he determined as the 'internal systems' facing 'external systems' and the impact of systems or feedback loops on team dynamics and consequently the effectiveness of teams.

An example of a system is the water cycle. Water is condensed from the atmosphere into clouds. It falls onto the earth and is collected into some form of reservoir. Humans channel the water into homes, factories, buildings, etc. It is then utilised and transformed into waste water which travels into the rivers and seas to be evaporated back into the clouds, thus beginning the cycle all over again. At each stage, there are factors that influence the system, such as drought, overusage and contamination. Equally, social systems can be affected by political, economic, social or technological factors and therefore indicate the complexity and vulnerability of any system, as well as an ability to adapt to change. Understanding systems and how they work can have an impact on problem solving, team working and the management of change (see useful websites for more information on management application of systems thinking).

While the importance of Homans' focus on individuals in small groups is now less often quoted, the fundamental findings of his work help to illuminate the factors that influence small group functioning as a system and the consequences of those interactions, such as the impact of the manager's leadership style and external organisational infrastructures. Homans considered the essential elements of a group system to be the activities, processes, interactions, interpersonal relationships and attitudes of team members towards the goals of the team. See Figure 2.1 for a contemporary version of Homans' conceptual scheme.

The conceptual feedback loop scheme Homans designed can help us to analyse groups and pinpoint problem areas when teams are ineffective. The importance of this work is to acknowledge that each action has an effect on another part of the process in a system, which is a major characteristic of systems theory and also of any small group interaction. Homans' studies led to the development of social exchange theory and the premise that social interaction is based on the exchange of rewards.

Figure 2.1: Homans' (1961) conceptual scheme of a small social system modified to reflect external and internal influences on consequences or effective outputs of a team in the twenty-first century

Theory summary: Social exchange theory

This theory is predicated on establishing and sustaining reciprocity in social relationships, or mutual gratification between individuals, and the comparison of alternatives. The theory relies on the assumption that humans are rational and willing to exchange items, material or emotional, that are important to them for the benefit of other people. Integral concepts of the theory are the notions of justice and fairness. If the perceived costs of a relationship outweigh the benefits, the theory predicts that a person will leave the relationship. However, criticisms of the theory are that it favours an economic model whereby all human interaction is likened to a process of cost benefit analysis. Furthermore, there are opportunities for coercion and power tactics through the use of punishments and rewards if benefits are withdrawn. This is particularly evident in hierarchical or highly structured environments and groupings. The perceived effect of social obligations versus the amount of freedom of choice to exchange commodities can also negatively affect relationships. Understanding the intricacies of social exchange theory can help you understand social relationships in a team when some people are more willing to help others, for example. (See the useful websites listed at the end of the chapter for further information.)

Creating effective team working

There has been much emphasis in the management literature on team building activities to enhance team effectiveness by focusing on both task and relationship aspects of team working. The aims of team building are generally to:

- establish goals or specific objectives;
- clarify the values, purpose and functions of the team;
- allocate or re-allocate work roles and responsibilities;
- establish or revive communication patterns;
- clarify the group norms or expected behaviours of the team;
- identify the decision making processes, responsibilities and hierarchies to define inter team relationships.

Team building can be facilitated by outside intervention to analyse problems and breakdown in communications. Team building can also be used to help integrate individuals into teams, thereby creating effectiveness from the beginning of a team's lifetime. This may require funding and time away from the work situation. Alternatively, the team leader can undertake an analysis of the team's functioning if the team only needs fine tuning (see useful websites at the end of the chapter for team building ideas). Team leaders can undertake an objective observation of team activities and then take this to team meetings for an open and self aware evaluation and discussion. The team leader will need to take the emotional temperature of the team to decide if this will be appropriate.

There will need to be preliminary preparation for any team building exercise to analyse and define the problems. This involves four steps:

1. Gathering information through different means, such as individual interviews with the team, anonymous survey, focus groups and team meetings.
2. Identifying the team's strengths and areas for development.
3. Creating a plan of action to present to the team.
4. Identifying time to work on the issues identified in steps 1 and 2 above.

Background information can also be gathered about the structures of the organisation in which the team works, the current work climate or work ambience or culture (e.g. financial constraints, status consciousness), team goals, professional characteristics of the team's work settings (e.g. mental health, community nursing, interdisciplinary, stroke rehabilitation, infection control), extent to which members work as autonomous individuals that link to a team, if based in a unit or spread out over a geographical area, complexity of roles and responsibilities, problem solving styles, interpersonal relationships and relations with other groups in the organisation.

Sullivan and Decker (2009) suggest the following eight questions should be asked:

1. To what extent does the team accept the goals of the organisation?
2. What, if any, hidden agendas interfere with the team's performance?
3. How effective is the team leadership?

4. To what extent do team members understand and accept their roles and responsibilities?
5. How does the team make a decision?
6. How does the team handle conflict? Are conflicts dealt with through avoidance or denial, force, accommodation, compromise, competition or collaboration?
7. What personal feelings do members have about each other?
8. To what extent do members trust and respect each other?

You can see that many of these questions relate to the characteristics of an effective team discussed earlier in the chapter.

Strategies for managing team problems

We have discussed how to create effective team working, and we go into more detail by studying different styles of leadership and management elsewhere in this text. There are, however, a few pointers from Antai-Otong (1997) that it is worth considering at this stage. These are aimed at specific team problems in nursing that a team leader will need to consider.

If the member is not a team player:

- consider carefully whether or not you want the person on the team;
- interact with the member assertively;
- give the person an opportunity to provide feedback on problematic situations;
- if communication with other team members is part of the problem, speak to the person in a one-to-one;
- listen actively when the person speaks, assessing verbal and non-verbal messages to identify any underlying issues or anxieties;
- avoid blaming and shaming which tends to create defensiveness and arguments.

If the member seems to lack a sense of personal accountability:

- explain how failure to take responsibility affects the whole team (and give an example);
- without blaming or shaming provide feedback from all team members.

If the team lacks clear goals:

- brainstorm activity to clarify short-term goals and develop an action plan with the team;
- strive for consensus regarding mission and goals;
- define member responsibilities;
- determine resources to accomplish goals (e.g. staffing expertise, financial, administrator support, time and equipment);
- periodically review team progress and achievements.

If team roles and boundaries are unclear:

- clarify role boundaries with the team's input;
- define all roles in the team, including the leader's;
- periodically review team's staff or professional development needs.

Communication in the team

One of the most frequent causes of poor team work is failing communication. A major problem in busy units and departments is dealing with distractions if essential information is to be communicated. Most distractions are through sensory perceptions, such as poor lighting or background noise, talking, music, ringing phones and interruptions. Moving to a quieter environment or agreeing a time to speak when all parties can concentrate can help to minimise distractions. Anxieties around reporting, heavy workloads and keeping up to date can also be distracting.

Different levels of knowledge can create frustration between staff and misunderstandings over expectations if a standard of knowledge is not met. This requires a culture of openness in the team so that members feel free to ask questions and are not embarrassed to admit to not having specific information.

Good communication in teams requires a rhythm of reciprocation and team engagement. When spontaneous decisions have to be made individuals can feel left out of the loop. All organisational and planning decisions should be agreed by consensus. However, an understanding that in exceptional circumstances there may be no time to communicate should also be agreed. Building in protected time, or a mechanism, to debrief the team on situations that fall outside the usual can help.

Differences in perception can misrepresent messages. The same message can be distorted through a lens of individual biases and preconceptions, socio-cultural, ethnic and educational differences, ending up sounding very different from what was intended. Teams need to develop tolerance and awareness of individual perceptual filters.

Distress, anxiety, high emotional states and certain personality traits, such as neuroticism which is one of five key personality traits typified by excessive anxiety or indecision, can interfere with message communications. (If you are interested in finding out more about personality traits and identifying your own traits see useful websites at the end of the chapter.) Being only human means home life stresses may be brought to the workplace. Team members need to feel safe to express their anxieties and have support from colleagues and the leader. However, if the stresses are interfering with effective working, occupational health support should be sought.

Dealing with meetings and committees

When you have a busy day ahead with many things on your to-do list the last thing you may feel like spending time on is either going to a meeting or leading one. They have a reputation for being boring and ineffective. But to ensure everyone uses their time efficiently and purposively a well led meeting can produce some very satisfying results. Meetings are the processes by which organisations conduct their business through committee structures. There are different types of committees with distinct responsibilities and decision making powers. Formal committees that are part of the governance structures of an organisation have different levels of authority and scope to make decisions. The highest level of committee structure is Board level (see useful websites for further information). The responsibilities and functions of any committee are outlined in the Terms of Reference along with the membership, frequency and quorate requirements. Very often these committees will have sub committees that are convened to deal with specific tasks or matters that need specialist and focused attention.

Other committees may have an advisory remit but no authority or power although they may have a strong influence on decisions. Committees are also set up to undertake specific tasks to be completed in a defined time span. An example is to develop a proposal for service development. The committee may then be tasked with implementing the developments or alternatively charged with investigating problems that require recommendations to be sent to a formal committee for action. Another form of committee will monitor activities such as standards or quality enhancement.

At ward or unit level the team meetings, where staff get together to discuss issues and problems and formulate local policies and procedures, are the focal point of work life. These meetings need to be seen as the pivotal place for decisions, discussions and forward planning to enhance the work environment and service delivery. It is the team leader's responsibility to ensure that the relevance and role of the meetings is understood and valued by team members. It should also be a time to enjoy being with colleagues who have a shared vision of their working lives.

Preparation; place and time; participation

The key to successful meetings is to follow the 3 Ps; Preparation, Place and time, and Participation. *Preparation* is about clearly identifying the purpose of the meeting. Even if it is a short meeting there should be an agenda with items to be discussed plainly stated and an indication as to whether the item is for discussion, decision or information. The leader needs to think ahead about the agenda items and undertake pre-reading, be ready to respond to questions and have potential solutions to problems at the ready as well as an idea of delegated responsibilities if this is required.

Place and time: advance information about venue and duration are vital. Meetings are work and not social gatherings, so an emphasis on getting things done and an action orientated approach are needed to encourage effective use of time. Members will also think it worthwhile attending if their time is not wasted.

Participation: your knowledge of team dynamics and the roles your team members play, whether nurturing or task orientated, will be valuable in understanding how your team members will participate in the meeting. Their ability to contribute will also depend on their level of skills and knowledge. However, this could be detrimentally affected by the phenomenon known as **group think** and is a particular concern if you have a philosophy of self directedness in a group of experienced professionals. The ability to chair meetings, take notes if necessary, delegate activities and follow up on actions are key elements of an effective meeting.

Theory summary: From group think to team think

In the 1970s social psychologist Irving Janis identified the phenomenon of group think that happens when a group makes faulty decisions. This is due to pressures from within the group whose members ignore alternatives and make irrational decisions that

continued opposite...

continued...

ignore the humanising factors present in other groups or sections of an organisation or community. When group members are from the same background, are insulated from outside influences and there are no clear decision making structures, they are particularly susceptible to group think. There are eight documented symptoms of group think:

1. **An illusion of invulnerability,** which creates excessive optimism that encourages taking extreme risks.
2. **Belief in collective rationalisation,** in which members discount warnings and do not reconsider their assumptions.
3. **Belief in inherent morality,** in which members believe in the rightness of their cause and therefore ignore the ethical or moral consequences of their decisions.
4. **Stereotyped views of other groups,** leading to negative views of 'the enemy' which make effective responses to conflict seem unnecessary.
5. **Direct pressure on dissenters,** involves putting members under pressure to avoid expressing arguments against any of the group's views.
6. **Self-censorship,** meaning that doubts and deviations from the perceived group consensus are not expressed.
7. **Illusion of unanimity,** in which the majority view and judgements are assumed to be unanimous.
8. **Self-appointed 'mind guards'** involves members protecting the group and the leader from information that is problematic or contradictory to the group's cohesiveness, view and/or decisions.

When groups are tightly knit and under pressure to make decisions, irrational decisions are likely as the group does not consider alternatives. This leads to carelessness and a need to achieve unanimity. The overall outcome is groups who have a low probability of successful decision making.

To move towards 'team think', team leaders need to facilitate discussions in teams that are not reliant only on members of the team, by introducing observers to the team or other specialists to give a point of view. Dealing with dominant members, as discussed previously, and not putting the team under pressure will also offset these effects. One of the main factors is to always consider alternative perspectives and the viewpoints or goals of other teams or activities in the organisation to gain a wider viewpoint of how decisions fit into the whole picture before making final decisions.

Interdisciplinary team working

Up till now this chapter has focused on team working within a professional group or disciplinary area, although it is acknowledged that there are many different types of teams working within the four fields of nursing: adult, mental health, child health and learning disabilities. In healthcare today there is an increasing need for professionals from different disciplines to work together to improve patient services for seamless care. Nurses, physicians, dieticians, social workers, pharmacists, physiotherapists, administrators and technicians may all find themselves working together with a common aim but a different perspective on how to achieve this aim.

Activity 2.4   *Evidence-based practice and research*

In your most recent practice placement, were you aware of any interdisciplinary teams functioning in the organisation? Next time you are in practice ask your mentor if there are any interdisciplinary teams and find out what the objectives are for these teams. Next, go to the Department of Health website and search for the document 'Health and Social Care Policy and the Interprofessional Agenda'. Read through the document to find the three competencies identified as key to interdisciplinary team working. Discuss with your mentor if the teams identified in your practice area are addressing these core competencies.

At the beginning of this chapter, the NMC Standards Domain Leadership, management and team working, competency 7, sets out specifically nurses' requirements for interdisciplinary working. Use this as a guide to analyse one interdisciplinary team's activity in your placement area. You may want to make notes for your assessment portfolio.

An outline answer to this activity can be found at the end of the chapter.

According to Hewison and Sim (1998) interprofessional working requires co-operation and mutual understanding, yet there are many barriers that can prevent this from happening. They explored the role of professional codes of ethics and the potential to foster professional distinctiveness and exclusivity. By identifying areas of common ground, in particular around 'whistle blowing', they felt multi-disciplinary working could develop. To achieve effective interprofessional working they argued that the role of management was crucial in leading teams in order to minimise professional rivalries and retain a central focus on patient need.

The following is an account of a study to examine the effectiveness of a team and the multi-disciplinary working processes.

Research summary: The impact of team processes on psychiatric case management

This is a study undertaken to identify the structures and interactions within community mental health teams that facilitate or impede effective teamwork and psychiatric case management. The view of the researchers was that effective case management requires close collaboration between case managers or care co-ordinators and other members of the multi-disciplinary mental health team, yet there has been little research into this relationship. A multiple case study of seven UK community mental health teams was conducted between 1999 and 2001, using qualitative methods of participant observation, semi-structured interviews and document review. Factors were identified from the study that impacted on the ability of care co-ordinators to act effectively. These were 'structure

continued opposite...

continued...

and procedures'; 'disrespect and withdrawal'; 'humour and undermining'; 'safety and disclosure'.

Care co-ordination was enhanced when team structures and policies were in place and where team interactions were respectful. Where members felt disrespected or undermined, communication, information sharing and collaboration were impaired, with a negative impact on the care provided to service users. The researchers concluded that teams require clear operating procedures alongside trust and respect across the professions, if there is to be open, safe and reflective participation.

Chapter summary

This chapter has given you an overview of how teams work and how you might better undestand the way in which individuals in teams work together. There are strategies in the chapter to help you work more effectively with others in a leadership capacity or collegeate manner in teams. The chapter has only touched the surface and you are strongly recommended to access the useful websites or further reading to provide you with more detailed guidance.

Activities: Brief outline answer

Activity 2.4 (page 34)

Health and Social Care Policy and the Interprofessional Agenda, page 7

www.dh.gov.uk/prod_consum_dh/groups/dh_digitalassets/documents/digitalasset/dh_078444.pdf (accessed 17 March 2011)

Three clusters of competencies:

1. Personal competences: learning to learn; team working; networking; creativity; entrepreneurship; leadership; defining a project.

2. Technical competences: PC user; Internet user; telecommunications user; environment-friendly behaviour.

3. Theoretical competences: foreign languages; European and global citizenship; scientific developments; understanding cultural diversity.

Further reading

Bach, S and Grant, A (2011) *Communication and Interpersonal Skills* (2nd edition). Exeter: Learning Matters.
Two chapters deal with effective team working and the working environment – Chapter 5: Understanding Potential Barriers; and Chapter 7: The Environmental Context.

Goodwin, B and Clemow, R (2010) *Nursing and Interprofessional Practice* (2nd edition). Exeter: Learning Matters.

Chapter 6: Teamwork is entirely written about interdisciplinary team work.

Useful websites

www.acas.org.uk/index.aspx?articleid=1218

Advisory, Conciliation and Arbitration Service (ACAS) dealing with conflict at work.

www.managementhelp.org/grp_skll/meetings/meetings.htm

Free Management Library information on preparing, planning, leading and evaluating meetings.

www.bbc.co.uk/labuk/experiments/personality

Personality Traits – the big five BBC self test and information on the latest meta theory of personality.

http://managementhelp.org/systems/systems.htm#anchor6759

Free Management Library on the development and application of systems theory to analyse problems and influence change management.

www.businessballs.com/teambuilding.htm

This site provides ideas for team building and also discussion around corporate social responsibility and ethical organisations.

www.belbin.com

Home page for Belbin's team role theory, role descriptors and explanations of the theory.

www.infed.org/thinkers/george_homans.htm
www.angelfire.com/bug/theory_project/Exchange_Theory.htm

These two websites both provide background to the work of the sociologist George Homans and the development of Social Exchange Theory.

Chapter 3
Working with individuals in teams

NMC Standards for Pre-registration Nursing Education

This chapter will address the following competencies:

Domain 1: Professional values

6. All nurses must understand the roles and responsibilities of other health and social care professionals, and seek to work with them collaboratively for the benefit of all who need care.

Domain 3: Nursing practice and decision making

10. All nurses must evaluate their care to improve clinical decision making, quality and outcomes, using a range of methods, amending the plan of care, where necessary, and communicating changes to others.

Essential Skills Clusters

This chapter will address the following ESCs:

Cluster: Organisational aspects of care

12. People can trust the newly registered graduate nurse to respond to their feedback and a wide range of other sources to learn, develop and improve services.

14. People can trust the newly registered graduate nurse to be an autonomous and confident member of the multi-disciplinary or multi agency team and to inspire confidence in others.

15. People can trust the newly registered graduate nurse to safely delegate to others and to respond appropriately when a task is delegated to them.

16. People can trust the newly registered graduate nurse to safely lead, co-ordinate and manage care.

17. People can trust the newly registered graduate nurse to work safely under pressure and maintain the safety of service users at all times.

19. People can trust the newly registered graduate nurse to work to prevent and resolve conflict and maintain a safe environment.

Chapter aims

After reading this chapter, you will be able to:

*   understand the significance of the concepts 'responsibility' and 'accountability' in relation to individuals in teams;

continued overleaf...

continued...

- evaluate the factors affecting the delegation of work to others in a team;
- evaluate the role of personal development plans for an individual in a team;
- understand the relevance of individual, organisational, generational and cultural differences to team working.

Introduction

In this chapter topics such as individual roles, responsibility and accountability with reference to the NMC Code of Professional Conduct will be discussed along with techniques for delegating. Personal development plans, performance appraisal and staff development principles will be explored. Cultural and generational differences will be discussed. Employment issues such as health and safety legislation and risk management will be included in this chapter. How to recruit, select and retain staff to work in teams will be covered briefly in Chapter 7. In addition, you will find it helpful to look at the NMC (2008) Code of Professional Conduct, which has specific guidance for nurses and midwives working in teams. Three key areas are covered in this guidance:

1. Share information with your colleagues.
2. Work effectively as part of a team.
3. Delegate effectively.

Activity 3.1	*Evidence-based practice and research*

Go to the NMC web page and review the underpinning principles of these the three themes proposed by the NMC.

These principles and themes are further discussed throughout this chapter.

The 2010 NMC Standards for Pre-registration Nursing Education and the NMC Code of Professional Conduct place considerable emphasis on team working and the responsibility of both the individual in the team and the team leader. In this chapter we will be focusing on the leadership role in supporting individuals in the team.

Individual roles, responsibility and accountability

In the previous chapter we looked at the many different forms and types of team and the ways in which teams can work together. In this chapter we will be concentrating on the individuals in the team and begin by looking at roles and responsibilities. Each team will have a defined purpose indicated in the two scenarios below.

Scenarios: Different examples of teams

Team A is brought together for a short-term activity such as the length of a shift. This could be a band 5 nurse caring for six patients in a section of a ward with possibly, and depending on the acuity of the needs of the patients or the seriousness of the illnesses, another band 5 colleague and two healthcare assistants from 7 a.m. till 3 p.m.

Team B is a multi-disciplinary team convened to work together for a longer duration to implement a new service initiative to improve patient care. In this example it is a project group to ensure patients receive dignified care on mixed sex wards.

Within each of these teams an individual team member will have a role or a part to play in completing a task and the overall remit of the team and be responsible for various actions. It is worth reminding ourselves of the meaning of the word 'responsible' and how that relates to the concept of accountability.

Activity 3.2   *Critical thinking*

Write out your definitions of 'responsible' and 'accountable' without referring to a dictionary. Think about what the differences are between the two concepts.

Then think about what the difference is for those who are leading teams and for those who are being led. The exercise should be about leadership styles and priorities, not accountability, etc.

Further guidance is given on this activity at the end of the chapter.

The next step is to ensure that team members understand their responsibilities in a task. A team leader is expected to assign responsibility for activities and this can become a minefield of emotions and hurt feelings if communicated inappropriately or to a person with the wrong skill set or knowledge. We will discuss this in more detail later in the chapter under the heading of delegation, but in this discussion we are focusing on conveying a sense of responsibility to complete team work successfully. This is not achieved by magic or guesswork or estimates of a team member's capabilities. It requires some clear thinking about what is expected, clear communication and checking progress throughout the task. If this is not done, leaders are responsible for less than satisfactory results and cannot hold team members accountable for any shortfalls. To ensure responsibilities are understood and carried out:

* identify the appropriate team member with the skills and knowledge to carry out the task in the team;
* ensure resources are available for the task to be completed or advise the team member how to obtain resources;
* explain and assign the task;
* identify the level of support to be given to the team member (e.g. are they novice or experienced?);

- set the standards;
- check progress.

Make sure the standards are met and the task completed also.

Delegation

As a team leader you can only delegate those tasks for which you are responsible. As we have seen in the discussion above and in the activity, the delegator remains accountable for the task, whereas the delegate is accountable to the delegator and has responsibilities for the task being assigned.

Delegation is a means of dividing up the workload in a team. It is also a way to help others develop or enhance their abilities and skills. It can promote team working, foster collaboration and increase the amount of work achievable in a given time when compared with a person working alone.

Delegation is not a means of escaping tasks or responsibilities that you do not want. Nor is it work or task allocation. Allocating tasks is to transfer a task from one person to another, whereas delegation gives someone the authority to carry out a task in place of the person who would normally undertake that task. By transferring authority, the person has the right to act and is empowered to undertake the task (i.e. this could be to ask others to undertake sub tasks as part of the overall activity). This difference should be made explicit to the delegate when a task is delegated.

Case studies

Let's return to the scenario of team B. Within this group there are representatives from different wards in a hospital as the initiative is to be undertaken across the organisation. The team also includes representatives of different disciplines. Once a plan of action has been agreed to ensure dignity is implemented on the wards, the representatives will go back to their bases and initiate changes in the ward to bring about a successful outcome. They will need the collaboration of their peers, subordinates and, possibly, superiors to carry out sub tasks. They may be experts in change management strategies and be able to charm the birds from the trees, but they will also need the authority to undertake this task and have that recognised by the teams they are going to be working with. Multi-disciplinary workers may have to work with professions other than their own. To be successful, they will also need their personal skills and the support of the authority invested in the group to bring about these changes. The authority invested in the project group, probably by a senior member of the Directorate or Division, will provide the legitimate authority for the project to carry out adjustments in the wards.

In the case of team A, where tasks are being divided amongst the team, the aim is to assign relevant activities to the appropriately qualified, or grade of, staff. The team leader will have the authority to assign the tasks and the responsibility to match activities to grade or competence. However, the team member has the responsibility for their own activities and the care of the patient.

Delegation decisions

Who to delegate to and how to delegate are, for the novice, quite daunting decisions. There are several potential competing thoughts and feelings impacting these decisions, such as:

- guilt in asking someone else to do a job that you are well qualified or competent to undertake;
- reluctance to delegate if you think you can do a task better or quicker;
- having to ask someone you are equal to in grade or who you haven't worked with before.

Activity 3.3   *Reflection*

Take a moment to think of any other obstacles that may inhibit you delegating or that you have observed in your placement experiences. Think about this from the point of view of both the delegator and the delegate.

Further guidance is given on this activity at the end of the chapter.

Working with skill mix

The changing workforce today means that **skill mix** in teams, with different grades working together, is increasing. In NHS acute care settings, increasing numbers of healthcare assistants (HCAs) will be working alongside qualified nurses undertaking whole patient care and not just tasks such as observations of temperature, pulse and respirations (Gainsborough, 2009). The majority of HCAs are employed on band 3 grades and you may want to request a copy of the generic job description (JD) for this grade to understand the scope of practice for this grade. The JD should link to the NHS Agenda for Change (AfC) band and the NHS Knowledge and Skills framework national clinical grading criteria. Some HCAs will take up Assistant or Associate Practitioner (AP) roles, with many having completed a specialised Foundation Degree in healthcare. These were introduced by the Skills for Health organisation in 2000. HCAs with this specialist qualification can move from the AfC band 3 grade to band 4. It would be worth your while looking at what the difference is in these two grades and the difference in the roles and responsibilities of an AP and a registered practitioner. As a recap, the table below outlines the current AfC bands for all NHS employees. Each band has a corresponding pay scale, the details of which can be found on the Agenda for Change website (listed at the end of this chapter).

Band 1	Administration, catering, domestic, portering
Band 2	Administration, catering, clinical support worker, patient transport, pharmacy assistant
Band 3	Microbiology assistant, secretary, security, emergency care support workers, occupational therapy assistants, physiotherapy assistants, speech therapy assistants, nursing assistants

continued overleaf...

continued...

Band 4	Mortuary, radiography or occupational therapy assistant, office manager, medical secretary, operating department practitioner (during training or entry level), assistant psychologists, nursing auxiliaries and nursery nurses, ambulance practitioners, physiotherapy assistants, speech therapy assistants
Band 5	Nurse & midwife (old D and E grades), dental technician (entry level), diagnostic/therapeutic radiographers, dietician, occupational therapist, paramedic, emergency medical technician, senior pharmacy technician, physiotherapist, assistant psychologists (higher grade), clinical physiologists, operating department practitioner (qualified), speech & language therapists (newly qualified)
Band 6	Junior sister/specialist senior staff nurse, senior II radiographer (diagnostic/therapeutic), art therapist, specialist dental technician, paramedic practitioner, emergency nurse/care practitioner, health visitor, nurse specialist, trainee clinical psychologist, pharmacist, senior clinical physiologists, senior physiotherapist
Band 7	Senior sister, senior radiographer (diagnostic/therapeutic team leader), chief dental technician, management – clinical & administrative, qualified psychologist, specialist pharmacist, chief clinical physiologists, senior physiotherapist
Band 8	Advanced pharmacists, nurse & midwife consultants, superintendent radiographers (diagnostic/therapeutic), higher management, psychologists, senior therapists (divided into four bands – a, b, c, d), senior chief clinical physiologists, consultant psychologists who run large services, chief pharmacists managing large/multiple departments

Table 3.1: Agenda for Change bands

Sources: DH (2004) and the document DH_4090843 from the Department of Health website.

In addition, some HCAs will have achieved National Vocational Qualifications (NVQs) at level 3 or 4. NVQs are a competency based qualification and there are five levels. Although NVQs are not usually compared directly to conventional academic qualifications, approximate equivalences have been established (see Table 3.2). Additionally, NVQ's are currently in the psocess of being replaced by the new Qualifications Credit Framework (QCF). See the weblink on page 54 for more information

NVQ Level	**Equivalent education level**
Level 1 Competence that involves the application of knowledge in the performance of a range of varied work activities, most of which are routine and predictable	Foundation General National Vocational Qualification, three to four GCSEs at grades D–E, Business & Technology Education Council (BTEC) first certificate

— continued opposite...

continued...

Level 2 Competence that involves the application of knowledge in a significant range of varied work activities, performed in a variety of contexts. Collaboration with others, perhaps through membership of a work group or team, is often a requirement	Five GCSEs at grades A*–C, BTEC first diploma
Level 3 Competence that involves the application of knowledge in a broad range of varied work activities performed in a wide variety of contexts, most of which are complex and non-routine. There is considerable responsibility and autonomy and control or guidance of others is often required	Two or more A levels, BTEC Ordinary National Diploma (OND), City & Guilds Advanced Craft
Level 4 Competence that involves the application of knowledge in a broad range of complex, technical or professional work activities performed in a variety of contexts and with a substantial degree of personal responsibility and autonomy. Responsibility for the work of others and the allocation of resources is often present	BTEC Higher National Certificate (HNC) or Higher National Diploma (HND), or City & Guilds Full Technological Certificate/Diploma
Level 5 Competence that involves the application of a range of fundamental principles across a wide and often unpredictable variety of contexts. Very substantial personal autonomy and often significant responsibility for the work of others and for the allocation of substantial resources features strongly, as do personal accountabilities for analysis, diagnosis, design, planning, execution and evaluation	National Qualifications Framework levels, ordinary degree levels 5–6

Table 3.2: Comparison of NVQ and National Education Certificates and Awards

Source: Information compiled from the Directgov – Education and Learning website (see page 53 for address).

In skill mix teams providing acute care to adult patients qualified nurses will need to delegate care to HCAs and other non-professionally registered staff such as domestic or ancillary personnel. In community settings health visitors delegate care to nursery nurses and band 5 nurses (staff nurses) who undertake some developmental screening. In some teams, such as intermediate care in the community, community practitioners are band 5 staff nurses working with community specialist practice home nurses. In acute mental health settings assistant practitioners work with registered mental health nurses. In child care nursery nurses work with staff nurses and in learning disability settings registered learning disability nurses work with nursing assistants.

Enabling staff development through delegation

By delegating tasks and responsibilities to other members of the team, opportunities can be provided for staff development, increased job satisfaction and promotion. However, certain factors have to be considered such as the need for a positive organisational culture that encourages delegation, personal qualities that engender co-operation and a willingness to collaborate, the appropriate resources (equipment and learning environment), and appropriate supervision or guidance for the task.

Selecting the right person to delegate to requires a corresponding leadership style. It is often assumed that delegation is a management role; however, recognising the talents and strengths of individuals and working with their singular developmental stages requires leadership qualities. Kotter (1990) recognised this and developed a scheme for matching the appropriate leadership style to the individual's levels of commitment and competence. This enables a leader to draw out the best in their team members and identify where development needs to take place. Table 3.3 outlines an adaptation of Kotter's ideas. We discuss coaching in Chapter 5.

Developmental level of individuals	Appropriate leadership style
Low competence – High commitment	Directing
Some competence – Low commitment	Coaching
High competence – Variable commitment	Supporting
High competence – High commitment	Delegating

Table 3.3: Matching individual levels of competence and motivation for tasks with leadership style

Source: Adapted from Kotter (1990).

Personal development plans

We have just talked about developing staff, so it would seem timely to introduce the topic of development planning. The personal development plan (PDP) (sometimes called individual development plan or staff review) is intended to help employees enhance existing skills or knowledge and develop new skills to fulfil an existing role. If responsibilities have increased the PDP may be utilised to identify a level that requires a re-grading to a higher grade. Alternatively, it can be used to identify a role at a grade equivalent to a previous role. In NHS settings the PDP should be carried out annually and is a method of ensuring staff maintain their skills and knowledge to perform their roles.

The PDP provides a framework for:

- prioritising developmental support;
- planning the related activities, such as attending study days, seminars or courses, in an appropriate sequence and within agreed timescales;
- monitoring progress within those timescales;
- evaluating outcomes in terms of skills, knowledge and expertise;
- developing individual career plans and identifying organisational succession plans.

A specifically designed e-platform for working with PDPs in healthcare settings can be found on the Knowledge Skills Framework website. As a student you may have completed a PDP that looks at your personal growth and development during your course. As a newly qualified nurse you will be expected to follow a period of preceptorship which will give you an opportunity to identify areas you want to concentrate on during your preceptorship to extend your confidence in specific skills and knowledge. As you progress in experience and seniority you may be involved in undertaking PDPs for HCAs and you would be advised to look out for any training being offered as each organisation has a slightly different emphasis on how they conduct the PDP process. As a registered practitioner you will be required to maintain your professional knowledge to remain on the NMC register. Known as PREP (Post Registration Education and Practice), you are required to declare you have completed the following every three years:

* 450 hours of registered practice in the previous three years;
* 35 hours of learning activity (Continuing Professional Development) in the previous three years.

The practice element can be met through administrative, supervisory, teaching, research and managerial roles as well as providing direct patient care.

Activity 3.4	*Research and reflection*

Go to the resources section in this chapter and follow the link to the NMC web pages for PREP. Take a look at the PREP handbook and consider how you will maintain your portfolio of activities to ensure your professional registration is up to date once you are qualified.

As this answer is based on your own observation, there is no outline answer at the end of the chapter.

Performance appraisal

Redshaw (2008) investigated the role and extent of appraisal in nursing. At the time only six out of ten staff in the NHS received a formal appraisal. There is a distinction between appraisal – which is the judgement and assessment of the worth or value of an employee's performance at work – and personal development – which is a process of mutually planning (between staff member and senior staff in the organisation) supporting activities for an individual to undertake their role in the workplace. Appraisal does not always have a good press as staff can feel that it is a waste of time or does not measure accurately their contribution to the work. Alternatively, some staff want to know how they are performing and have some measure of performance as a yardstick to improve, for their own satisfaction or to progress in their career or work roles. Chapter 7 gives more information about performance appraisal.

There are different forms of appraisal scheme: top down (the most common), self-appraisal and peer appraisal, upward appraisal where appraiser reports on management's performance (the least common) and multi-rater appraisal which is usually in the form of 360 degree feedback about an individual from a variety of peers, subordinates, external and internal appraisers and superiors.

There are difficulties with performance appraisal both in the implementation and management of appraisal schemes. Some appraisal systems can be time consuming both for the interview and the form completion. The objective of appraisal is to identify and reward performance. If this is not achieved in practice the scheme will lack commitment. If there is an appraisal system alongside a development planning scheme the allocation of rewards can undermine the personal developmental aspects as the emphasis will be on the organisational aims and outputs. There are also concerns about the subjectivity of making appraisals that can be influenced by personal attributes of the appraiser or employee and environmental or situational factors such as individual health or organisational changes.

Support for staff – including performance review – can raise standards in the workplace. However, the quest for better performance has not always been accompanied by a better system of appraisal. According to Redshaw (2008), most important process for improved performance is not to set goals and order staff to achieve them, but to improve relationships in which they are highly valued and have a sense of belonging. So, the development of positive manager/employee relationships is an effective way to improve the appraisals process. Conflicts, lack of understanding of the aims of the process and mutual distrust will have a negative effect, resulting in staff finding it difficult to accept criticism and feedback. This in turn will have a wider impact on staff performance. This is especially relevant in team-based work where the style of the leader can influence colleagues' performance and attitudes towards appraisal. Another factor is the way in which feedback is handed to employees. Giving feedback can be challenging and managers need good communication skills to ensure feedback is constructive and helpful. Feedback that is focused on blame damages self-confidence, whereas constructive criticism to recognise and improve poor performance is appropriate.

Case study: Ensuring adequate nutrition

The setting is a busy acute female medical ward. In a six bedded bay, Mary, a slight 72-year-old who was originally admitted with unstable type 2 diabetes, is waiting to be discharged home. Although the ward staff have told her she won't be leaving until after lunch, Mary has had her bags packed since 7 a.m. as she is keen to leave the ward. Mary is a quiet and undemanding person who rarely complains. The band 5 team leader for the shift, Sandy, passes by the bed and sees that Mary has been provided with her lunch of soup and a sandwich. Nutrition is an important part of Mary's recovery plan to treat her diabetes and also to help her restore her weight which is currently below her expected Body Mass Index (BMI). Mary should be having fortified soups and not the usual soup from the hospital menu. Fortified soups are available for patients in the ward kitchen. Sandy has spoken to the HCAs and ward hostess before about ensuring that Mary has fortified soups and that she receives reinforcing messages when she has her meals of the relevance and importance of maintaining her nutrition once she is at home. Sandy believes the HCAs are capable of giving health education as well as ensuring patients receive the appropriate nutrition. This would be in line with the NHS Knowledge and Skills Framework (KSF) section on Health and Wellbeing and appropriate for the role of an HCA to undertake. She also believes that the HCA, Joanna in this case, should have responsibility for ensuring the ward hostess provides the correct soup and that Joanna should monitor this. Sandy resolves to speak to the HCA to provide feedback on her performance and what she expects the HCA's role to be in this respect.

Fowler (1996) suggests the following principles when giving feedback:

1. Be specific and give examples.
2. Be constructive and focus on what can be learnt from the event.
3. Avoid comments about attitude or personality that cannot realistically be changed and concentrate on behaviour and the way it affects performance.
4. Give feedback regularly and do not wait for annual reviews; it should be timely and as close to the event as possible.
5. Encourage self-reflection – feedback is not just about telling.
6. Avoid argument – a practical discussion about differences of opinion on performance is much more helpful. Listen to the other person's point of view.
7. Explain the reasons for the request for a change that may be needed and encourage the development of an action plan.
8. Take feedback yourself – the discussion should be two-way and there may be lessons to learn from your own performance.
9. Encourage openness and this will lead to the other person seeking regular feedback as part of the culture of the unit/department and your leadership style.

Activity 3.5 — *Decision making*

Imagine that you are Sandy, the band 5 staff nurse on this shift, who is leading the team. Make a draft plan of how you would give feedback to Joanna. What points would you make? What would be the principles upon which you would base your feedback for Joanna? When would you go about giving the feedback?

Further guidance is given on this activity at the end of the chapter.

Individual, cultural and generational differences

Working with individuals in teams, the team leader will encounter individual differences in the team members that have to be acknowledged and worked with to ensure effective working relationships. In Chapter 1, we examined different roles that individuals assume in a team by individual differences. The chapter concentrates on the individual traits and personality that a person has. In Chapter 2, we had a brief look at these characteristics and now we can further explore personal characteristics that fall within the 'Big Five Personality Theory'.

Research summary: Five Factor Model of Personality

In 1991 Barack and Mount reported on a study that they undertook to examine the relationships between workplace roles and individual personality characteristics defined in the 'Big Five Personality Theory' or Five Factor Model of Personality as it is known theoretically. The personality dimensions are: Extraversion, Emotional Stability,

continued overleaf...

continued...

Agreeableness, Conscientiousness, and Openness to Experience. These were matched to three job performance criteria (job proficiency, training proficiency and personnel data – i.e. age, time in occupation, etc.) for five occupational groups (professionals such as teachers, nurses and doctors; police; managers; sales; skilled/semi-skilled occupations).

The results of their analysis indicated that one dimension of personality, Conscientiousness, showed consistent relations with all job performance criteria for all occupational groups. For the remaining personality dimensions, the correlations varied by occupational group and professional criteria.

Extraversion was a valid predictor for two occupations involving social interaction: managers and sales (across criterion types). Also, both Openness to Experience and Extraversion were valid predictors of the training proficiency criterion (i.e. those persons who had a role as educators and this was across all professions in the study). Other personality dimensions were also found to be valid predictors for some occupations and some criterion types, but the correlation between the occupation and criterion was small (page 10).

Overall, the results illustrated the benefits of using the five-factor model of personality to predict suitability for job performance. The findings were thought to have numerous implications for research and practice, especially in the sub fields of personnel selection, training and development, and performance appraisal. This means that there is some substance to the theory that certain personal characteristics are better suited to certain occupational roles.

Organisational culture

Another factor to influence individual behaviour in teams is cultural mores. On one level this could be explored as the culture of the organisation. The philosophies and social and historical background to an organisation all shape the prevailing culture. In addition, practices within an organisation that are derived from leadership or management style also have an impact. For example, whether or not an organisation is people or task orientated, if there is an emphasis on control and command, the extent of tolerance to risk taking, if there is a reward culture or a blame culture, the manner in which an organisation responds to change – rapidly or at the pace of a snail – and finally the extent to which an individual willingly signs up to the philosophy of the organisation.

Activity 3.6 *Reflection*

Take a moment to reflect on the culture of the organisation you have worked in, or had practice experience in, most recently. Can you recognise any of the characteristics mentioned above? Then think about what kind of culture you would want to foster if you were leading a team.

As this answer is based on your own observation, there is no outline answer at the end of the chapter.

Cultural diversity

The other aspect of culture is the sociological phenomenon of culture, which affects our lives in a complex and multifaceted manner in our culturally diverse society. To work collaboratively in teams, nurses have to understand and respect unfamiliar behaviour patterns and attitudes without dismissing or devaluing them. Yet, this diversity needs to be harnessed to be effective and to meet patients' needs. Bach and Grant (2011) consider the relevance of focusing on cultural diversity and communication as this is often the first barrier to overcome.

There are thought to be four cultural dimensions ↔ along which cultures differ in the workplace:

- Directness – getting to the point ↔ implying the messages.
- Hierarchy – following orders ↔ engaging in debate.
- Consensus – dissenting is accepted ↔ unanimity is needed.
- Individualism – individual winners are acceptable ↔ team effectiveness is paramount.

Different attitudes to authority, culturally embedded notions of authority and power, perceptions of gender stereotypes, and acceptance of directness or expectations of hidden meanings in communications – all influence these cultural dimensions. A team leader will need to be observant to recognise at which point of these dimensions individuals are expected to behave in the team and how each individual will be interpreting these dimensions – depending on their social cultural background and the norms they are accustomed to. In addition, the philosophy of the organisation and the nature of the tasks that are undertaken (e.g. the perceived status of those tasks) will have an influence.

Generational differences

Every generation is affected by the time in which they are growing up. Influences such as economic (e.g. post World War II thriftiness), political (e.g. Thatcherism and individualistic political policies), social events (Bob Geldof Live Aid concerts), feminist ideology and technological advances will play a significant part in forming the context for attitudes to be formed about work. While the cusp years can vary depending on the individual, here's how the generations are typically described:

- Traditionalists or Veterans: Born before 1946.
- Baby Boomers: Born between 1946 and 1964.
- Generation X: Born between 1965 and 1980.
- Generation Y or Millennials: Born after 1980.

Patterson (2005) has gathered together observations from her work as an organisational psychologist and the business management literature to assemble impressions of the main characteristics associated with generations since the early part of the last century.

Traditionalists (1925 to 1945)	Baby boomers (1946 to 1964)	Generation X (1965 to 1980)	Millennials (1981 to present)
Practical	Optimistic	Sceptical	Hopeful
Patient, loyal and hardworking	Teamwork and co-operation	Self-reliant	Meaningful work
Respectful of authority	Ambitious	Risk-taking	Diversity and change valued
Rule followers	Workaholic	Balances work and personal life	Technology savvy

Table 3.4: Defining work characteristics

Source: Adapted from Patterson (2005).

While not everyone will fall into a defined category, taking note of generational diversity is important as intergenerational conflict, or lack of understanding of different generational mores, can impede plans, team work and ideas for service improvement. For example, a baby boomer manager may not be familiar with social networking and the impact technologies have had on social relationships. The manager's ideas on how relationships are communicated and sustained might involve paper notices on notice boards, whereas the millennial team members will be likely to expect messages to be posted on a social networking site.

Research summary: Generational differences

Smola and Sutton (2002) surveyed 350 baby boomers and gen Xers in 1974 and 1999 and found an overall change in work values as generations matured, such as giving work a lower priority in life and placing less value on feeling a sense of pride at work. In particular, the younger women tend to more often question workplace expectations, such as long work hours or taking work home, and they are often more open about their parenting obligations and commitments. The study also found generational differences, for example, at gen Xers report less loyalty to their companies, wanting to be promoted more quickly and being more 'me-oriented' than baby boomers. It is suggested that such differences are, in part, accounted for by workers' values shifting as they age.

Working in teams can cause clashes between individuals in the workplace. Baby boomers, traditionalists, gen Xers and millennials all represent different cultural norms as far as respecting tradition, social manners, speaking frankly about personal issues and attitudes to hierarchy are concerned. The generations will respond to change in different ways – fear of change can be expressed in one way if it results from being too used to certain ways of doing things, and in another way completely if it results from immaturity and insecurity. Baby boomers may find traditionalists inflexible, and be themselves perceived as self-absorbed in return. Gen Xers, on the other hand, may find themselves criticised for being cynical and negative while seeing baby boomers as having their own conventional rigidity, and millennials as spoiled upstarts. Such clashes may be reduced if there are opportunities for facilitated discussion in team meetings, helping the various participants to explore the benefits and disadvantages of different approaches to working methods. A team leader will have the role of encouraging effective listening between team members, reducing ambiguity and misunderstandings, supporting the sharing of expertise and recognition of individuals' contributions to the team. It is helpful if the various generational groups can be encouraged to understand why each might respond in a particular fashion, and how patients might benefit in each case.

This approach is even more useful in interdisciplinary teams if misunderstandings are to be avoided. Team members can then work towards seeking a balance between building on traditional procedures and supporting newer ideas to blend the different work ethics of the generational groups.

According to Patterson (2005) effective, or similar, messages are for:

- Traditionalists: 'Your experience is respected' or 'It is valuable to hear what has worked in the past'
- Baby boomers: 'You are valuable, worthy' or 'Your contribution is unique and important to our success'.
- Gen Xers: 'Let's explore some options outside of the box' or 'Your technical expertise is a big asset'.
- Millennials: 'You will have an opportunity to collaborate with other bright, creative people' or 'You have really rescued this situation with your commitment'.

Chapter summary

This chapter has given you an overview of how teams work and how you might better understand the way in which individuals in teams work together. There are strategies in the chapter to help you work more effectively with others in a leadership capacity or collegeate manner in teams. The chapter has only touched the surface and you are strongly recommended to access the useful websites or further reading to provide you with more detailed guidance.

Activities: brief outline answers

Activity 3.2 (page 39)

The term 'responsible' can be understood from two perspectives:

1. Being the cause of something, usually something wrong or disapproved of.

2. Being accountable to someone for an action or the successful carrying out of a duty.

In a team, the team member has responsibility for carrying out an activity to the standard required by the team leader. To avoid perspective number 1 above, where misunderstandings, inaccuracies and disappointments may have occurred, the required standard should be explained to the person who has the responsibility for the task. In this situation it is the team leader's responsibility to be clear about what is expected in a task and the team member's responsibility to accomplish the task. Spending time explaining to a team member what is required can save time later and also enable the team member to carry out the task up to the level required. It may be a peer who is in the team and in this case it would be helpful to clarify that both of you are working towards the same goal or outcome. If it is a subordinate or someone with untested skills or knowledge of the situation, an example or demonstration may be necessary to indicate the standard required for the task.

The term 'accountable' can also be understood from two perspectives:

1. The obligations to report, explain or justify a behaviour or activity that has taken place and take responsibility for this activity being carried out. In this sense a person is answerable to, or responsible to, another person, organisation or professional body for the manner in which an activity has been undertaken. A key factor here is the word obligation which can be interpreted as the legal responsibility or employment responsibility of the grade in which a person is employed. In this sense it is accepting ownership for the results, or lack thereof.

2. The capability of explaining why something has taken place (i.e. to give an account of something with reasons and/or evidence).

In nursing we more often use the first perspective rather than the second perspective as the concept of accountability is blended with responsibility. Therefore, the team leader is both accountable to the employer with the responsibility for carrying out the task through the activities of the team members. The team members are accountable to the team leader and have responsibility to them to carry out the required activity. However, the second perspective may be drawn upon if a person is required to give an account of the failure or success of a task.

Activity 3.3 (page 41)

Delegator
- Beliefs: lack of trust or confidence, believing others are incapable, belief that you are indispensable.
- Fears: fears of criticism, liability, blame for others' mistakes, loss of control, overburdening others, decrease in your own job satisfaction.
- Deficiencies: inexperience in delegation, organisational skills, ability to make decisions, knowledge of grade or competencies.

Delegate
- Beliefs: lack of confidence in own ability.
- Fears: of failure, being blamed for mistakes or incompetence, legal consequences.
- Deficiencies: overdependence on others in the team or superiors to shoulder responsibility, avoidance of responsibility.

Activity 3.5 (page 47)

What would be the points you would make?

1. Importance and rationale for nutrition in:
   a. diabetes type 2 treatment; and
   b. maintaining weight.

2. Importance of health education information about maintaining diet when patient goes home.

3. Ensure the ward hostess gives the correct type of soup to Mary by monitoring delivery.

4. Ensure Mary drinks the soup even though she is keen to go home and not make a fuss.

5. Has Joanna had any additional training in diet and nutrition, and in particular with type 2 diabetes? If not, is there a training day coming up soon that she could attend?

6. Is Joanna comfortable monitoring the ward hostess, and does she see this as part of her role and her work in the team on this section of the ward? If not, explain that you have this expectation and you will support Joanna to do this by mentioning this as the expectation for all HCAs in the next team meeting.

What would be the principles you would think of when giving Joanna feedback drawn from Fowler's (1996) list in the section on giving feedback in the text above?

When would you go about giving the feedback? It is suggested that feedback should be given at a time closest to the event occurring. You will have to balance this decision with an evaluation of the suitability of the time available either during a shift, or at the end of the shift, or at a pre-arranged time other than during the day of the shift. It depends on how busy you are and any other situational factors. However, do not let these factors obstruct you from your task. If this is the first time you are to give feedback you may want to let your ward manager know and practice how you are going to handle the situation with her/him. She/he can also give you support when the issue is raised in the team meeting.

Further reading

Bach, S and Grant, A (2011) *Communication and Interpersonal Skills for Nurses* (2nd edition). Exeter: Learning Matters.
An accessible introduction to the subject.

Sullivan, EJ and Decker, PJ (2009) *Effective Leadership and Management in Nursing* (7th edition). Harlow: Pearson International Edition. Chapter 10, Delegating Successfully.
Although this book is written for the USA the principles are transferable and this chapter provides some in-depth analysis of the difficulties and methods to overcome the art of delegation.

Useful websites

www.bbc.co.uk/labuk/experiments/personality/
Personality Traits – the big five BBC self test and information on the latest meta theory of personality.

www.e-ksfnow.org/New.htm
The website of the NHS Knowledge and Skills Framework.

www.dh.gov.uk/en/Publicationsandstatistics/Publications/PublicationsPolicyAnd Guidance/DH_4090843
Provides information on the Agenda for Change bands.

www.direct.gov.uk/en/EducationAndLearning/QualificationsExplained/DG_10039017
Government website explaining how the new QCF qualifications relate to NVQs and other qualifications.

www.dh.gov.uk/prod_consum_dh/groups/dh_digitalassets/@dh/@en/documents/ digitalasset/dh_4105472.pdf
Introduction to the NHS Knowledge and Skills Framework and its links to the NHS Agenda for Change National Pay Agreement.

http://rapidbi.com/created/personaldevelopmentplan.html# formonthejobdevelopmentrecord
This is a link to an example of a Personal Development Plan from a commercial organisation.

**www.nhsemployers.org/PayAndContracts/AgendaForChange/Pages/
Afc-AtAGlanceRP.aspx**
NHS Employers currently provides help and guidance on pay and employment issues in the NHS. It is a membership organisation of NHS trusts supported by the Department of Health.

www.nmc-uk.org/Documents/Standards/nmcPrepHandbook.pdf
Nursing and midwifery PREP requirements, as stated by the NMC.

**www.ofqual.gov.uk/qualification-and-assessment-framework/articles/145-explaining-
the-qualifications-and-credit-framework**
Website of the Qualifications and Curriculum Authority.

www.skillsforhealth.org.uk/getting-the-right-qualifications/vocational-qualifications
Skills for Health website giving information on QCF qualifications and foundation degrees.

Chapter 4
Conflict management and negotiation skills

NMC Standards for Pre-registration Nursing Education

This chapter will address the following NMC competencies:

Domain 1: Professional values

2. All nurses must practise in a holistic, non-judgmental, caring and sensitive manner that avoids assumptions, supports social inclusion; recognises and respects individual choice; and acknowledges diversity. Where necessary, they must challenge inequality, discrimination and exclusion from access to care.

Domain2: Communication and interpersonal skills

4. All nurses must recognise when people are anxious or in distress and respond effectively, using therapeutic principles, to promote their well-being, manage personal safety and resolve conflict. They must use effective communication strategies and negotiation techniques to achieve best outcomes, respecting the dignity and human rights of all concerned. They must know when to consult a third party and how to make referrals for advocacy, mediation or arbitration.

5. All nurses must use therapeutic principles to engage, maintain and, where appropriate, disengage from professional caring relationships, and must always respect professional boundaries.

Domain 4: Leadership, management and team working

4. All nurses must be self-aware and recognise how their own values, principles and assumptions may affect their practice. They must maintain their own personal and professional development, learning from experience, through supervision, feedback, reflection and evaluation.

Essential Skills Clusters

This chapter will address the following ESCs:

Cluster: Care, compassion and communication

1. As partners in the care process, people can trust a newly registered graduate nurse to provide collaborative care based on the highest standards, knowledge and competence.

continued overleaf...

• • *continued...* •

At entry to the register:

9. Is self aware and self confident, knows own limitations and is able to take appropriate action.

11. Acts as a role model in developing trusting relationships, within professional boundaries.

12. Recognises and acts to overcome barriers in developing effective relationships with service users and carers.

4. People can trust a newly qualified graduate nurse to engage with them and their family or carers within their cultural environments in an acceptable and anti-discriminatory manner free from harassment and exploitation.

At entry to the register:

6. Acts autonomously and proactively in promoting care environments that are culturally sensitive and free from discrimination, harassment and exploitation.

7. Manages and diffuses challenging situations effectively.

Cluster: Organisational aspects of care

19. People can trust the newly registered graduate nurse to work to prevent and resolve conflict and maintain a safe environment.

At entry to the register:

3. Selects and applies appropriate strategies and techniques for conflict resolution, de-escalation and physical intervention in the management of potential violence and aggression.

Chapter aims

After reading this chapter, you will be able to:

*   identify situations during which conflict might arise;
*   discuss strategies for preventing conflict arising;
*   demonstrate awareness of methods of managing conflict;
*   comment on your own ability to understand and manage yourself in difficult situations involving interpersonal conflict.

Introduction

Nursing involves caring for people during some of the most emotionally difficult times of their lives. As well as patients, nurses come into contact with relatives, friends and carers of patients who are themselves distressed and anxious. In some circumstances, nurses and other care staff can become upset or angry themselves.

Within any clinical setting there is the potential for anxiety, confusion, distress, hurt and pain to erupt into conflict. Sometimes distress arises as a result of a patient's physical condition.

At other times, frustration may surface as a result of apparent failures within systems, poor communication or lack of understanding.

Conflict may arise between patients and care staff; between patients; between care staff; between patients and significant others; or between staff and patients' significant others. Recognising the potential for conflict, learning how to prevent and how to manage conflict are all key skills in leadership and management. Perhaps the most important skill aspiring nurse leaders can have however is the ability to understand and manage themselves in such situations.

The purpose of this chapter is to enable you to explore some of the issues that contribute to the development of conflict in the clinical setting, and to examine strategies to prevent these occurring or to defuse such situations when they do occur.

What is conflict?

Understanding what conflict is and why it arises is fundamentally important in understanding both how to prevent it from occurring and how to manage it once it has arisen. Conflict is the expression of a disagreement between two or more parties that arises out of a difference in opinion, needs or desires between them. It is important to recognise that conflict is not usually about the individual him or herself; it is more likely to arise as a response to an individual's perception of a situation or circumstance. The prevention of conflict, therefore, has as much, if not more, to do with the management of perception as with anything else.

Not all conflict is physical in nature, although what started as a disagreement, a heated discussion or an argument can soon escalate to violence if it is not handled well. The following example encourages you to think through an everyday situation in a hospital to increase your understanding of how easily a confrontational situation can develop.

Case study: The protracted wait

Stan is a busy man who has to attend hospital regularly for monitoring of his emphysema. The hospital is quite old and Stan is forced to wait in the corridor along with the rest of the people attending the clinic because there is no waiting room. The corridor is cold and draughty, and has a constant stream of people through it. Stan has waited over an hour past his allotted appointment time and is fed up, not only with the hanging around but with having to sit in the corridor. Stan approaches the receptionist and demands to know how much longer he will have to wait. The receptionist's response while polite is not helpful as she does not know why the appointments are running so far behind. Stan is upset by the lack of information he is given and the seemingly poor communication within the team. He shouts at the receptionist for being 'incompetent'.

This case study illustrates how perception and the physical environment can contribute to bad feeling. Stan is aggrieved at having to wait in an environment that is not designed for the purpose for which it is being used. He is forced to wait for a protracted period of time but does not know why. When Stan tries to find out why he is waiting, he does not get what he considers to be a reasonable response. The receptionist is not being rude, but Stan's perception of the fact she is unable to give him a reason for the delay is that his needs are not being met and this is unacceptable.

We can imagine the same scenario acted out in various different ways which may lead to different outcomes. The receptionist might tell Stan to sit down and wait, thus escalating the situation to one of open conflict. She might apologise for the delay and say that she will find out what is happening and come back to him, thus meeting his need to feel that he is being taken seriously. She might empathise with Stan about his situation and say how bad it is for her as well; while this may distract Stan from shouting at her, it may lead to his anger being focused at other staff in the hospital. Evidently there may be little that she, or indeed many leaders or managers, can do about the physical surroundings (since this may require a considerable investment of money) but they can and must exercise control over the psychosocial, interpersonal, environment of care.

What is also clear from this scenario is that prevention of conflict is everyone's business. It may seem to some that it is the role of managers, senior staff and security to deal with issues of conflict when they arise. What the protracted wait scenario shows is this perception is wrong. Being polite and appearing to be helpful is the role of all staff whether they be care professionals, students or support workers. Clearly, and as is explored later in the chapter, one of the roles of the manager in this sort of scenario is to look for ways in which such situations can be better managed in the future to achieve better **outcomes** for patients.

Why managing conflict is important

The need to manage conflict effectively may seem obvious: conflict is just not nice. There are good reasons why managing conflict is important in the context of leadership and management, and these go beyond merely preventing an unpleasant situation.

The first reason that conflict management in care environments is important is it can negatively affect the experiences of patients and clients (Northam, 2009a). This applies equally to those involved in the conflict and those forced to witness it. The same is true of the staff in a department or team when conflict occurs regularly. The negative experiences of staff will almost certainly affect their ability to care and may give rise to absence through sickness associated with stress. Continued poor management of conflict may cause some staff to leave their posts, creating recruitment and retention issues.

Managing complaints and conflicts properly can lead to benefits for the team and the organisation. Recurrent complaints arising from the provision of care may be turned around to create opportunities for development. If conflict and complaints arise out of people's perceptions of the care they receive then these can be used to help redesign both the ways in which care is delivered and the nature of the care itself. A key message for leaders and managers in the management of conflict is therefore about learning from it. Properly managed, perhaps through the use of **clinical supervision** (see Chapter 5) and individual reflection (Hocking, 2006), conflict may prove to be a catalyst for innovation and creativity. **Total quality management** requires nurse leaders and managers to recognise and engage in practices which improve both the processes and practices of healthcare; this includes responding to complaints, criticism and compliments from clients.

While there is no specific legislation in the UK covering workplace conflict, bullying and the like, the Health and Safety at Work Act (1974) makes it quite plain that employers are responsible for the health of their employees – this includes their mental well-being. Legislation against discrimination on the grounds of age, sex, disability or ethnicity does exist and requires that managers behave in an equitable manner towards all of their employees (Equality Act, 2006) and that they protect employees from harassment in the workplace. This requires managers, leaders and all care staff to be aware of situations which might lead to conflict and to manage them and the behaviour of staff effectively.

Consider the following case study where conflict arising out of the way in which a service is provided is reflected on and used to develop a better way of working with potential to improve patients' experience.

Case study: The pain clinic

The pain clinic in the local district general hospital provides many services to local people, one of which is minor pain relieving procedures requiring a short period of sedation. Each morning ten people are admitted to the clinic to undergo procedures such as facet joint injections and selective nerve root blocks. Each procedure is quite short but requires a small amount of sedation so it usually takes about three hours to get through the whole procedures list.

Tom is asked to attend the clinic at 8 a.m. in order to have an injection to help manage his back pain. Tom duly arrives at 8 a.m. and sits in a waiting room along with the other nine people. By 9.30 a.m. Tom is still waiting to be admitted as he is the last on the procedures list for that day. Tom is irritated by the wait as he is in pain and the chairs in the waiting area are uncomfortable. He asks Emma, the nurse admitting the patients, why he has been brought in so early when it is clear he will not need to be in a bed until about 11 a.m.? Emma responds that is just the way the clinic runs. Tom protests loudly that this is silly and that there has to be a better way of running things. Another patient joins in saying they feel as if they are being treated like cattle being forced to wait for no apparent good reason. Both Tom and the other patient become quite excited and start to talk loudly about how ridiculous it all is until they are both called in to be admitted.

Emma is quite intimidated by what has happened. She reflects that this is a regular occurrence and perhaps the patients have a point about the way in which the clinic is run. She decides to talk to Hamida, the clinical nurse manager, about the complaints.

Hamida points out that the orthopaedic day unit in the same hospital sends out different appointments for admissions on surgery days, with an hour between patients. The staggered admission times mean one nurse can comfortably admit and prepare three or four people for surgery on the same day and no one is kept waiting unnecessarily. Emma reflects on this and decides she should go and see what the orthopaedic unit are doing to understand the pros and cons of their approach with a view to adopting the practice in the pain clinic.

What we can see in this case study is that patients have a real issue with being kept waiting, especially if they are in pain. Rather than ignoring this, hiding away or perhaps leaving the clinic, Emma takes on a leadership role and seeks to turn a problem into something that works for everyone's benefit. She reflects on the situation and then seeks help and support from a more experienced member of the team.

Perhaps the second key message of managing potential conflict is to listen to what is being said, rather than just to how it is being said. A third lesson might be to seek help in understanding and solving potential issues.

Again this case study shows the value of learning from and acting upon complaints to further improve the quality of care provision. If we can do this, we demonstrate our engagement, both as nurses and as leaders, with improving the lives of our patients.

Identifying potential sources of conflict

Conflict is a constant possibility in any organisation where there are human interactions (Johnson, 1994). The potential for conflict to arise in the hospital or other clinical setting is compounded by the type of work that occurs there. People visiting hospitals or other healthcare facilities, either as patients or visitors, are in physical and psychological distress. This means they are vulnerable, particularly if they do not understand what is happening. The fact that healthcare is often delivered in an autocratic manner also makes people feel vulnerable.

This vulnerability is perhaps not, in itself, something which nurses can eliminate. However, recognising it and doing something about it may make the difference between conflict arising or not. What is clear is that feeling vulnerable makes some people defensive and aggressive and in identifying this nurses, along with all care professionals, can do a lot to avert conflict.

Taking a leadership role in the management of conflict is every nurse's role. As we saw in the earlier chapter on the experience of leadership, this involves seeing the bigger picture and understanding how the structures within which we work affect both us and the people we work with. In good part these sentiments are reflected in the increasing importance of user consultation and patient involvement forums. Clearly the best way to understand how care is experienced is to ask the people experiencing it and the best way to improve how care is experienced is to again involve those in receipt of care.

It is worth reflecting on the effect a lack of understanding can have on how we feel about ourselves and others around us, and how this lack of understanding can create a real sense of vulnerability.

Activity 4.1   *Reflection*

Cast your mind back to your first day on your most recent clinical placement. Think about the feelings that you had about working in a team of people you did not know, in an area with which you were unfamiliar and with patients whose conditions you perhaps did not fully understand. Think about how all these unknowns made you feel. How did you react? Who made you feel less at ease? Who made you feel more at ease? What did people do that made you feel more or less at ease? What lessons can you draw from this experience to help you to understand how patients might feel and behave in unfamiliar circumstances?

There are some possible answers and thoughts at the end of the chapter.

This activity emphasises that fear is a natural response to the unknown, and what people do and say can have a great impact. Understanding what may create feelings of vulnerability in ourselves can help us to understand which issues might create vulnerability in others. Managing our encounters with others and recognising the potential for conflict that arises out of our interactions allows us to demonstrate the important, people-centred aspects of leadership.

The potential for conflict can be heightened by the amount of specialisation and organisational hierarchy that is present in many clinical teams (Swansburg and Swansburg, 2002) (for more on managing conflict in teams, see Chapter 2). The manner in which we choose to present ourselves to others can heighten feelings of inadequacy and fear. The specialist knowledge we have in an area and the position we hold can be used to create barriers between us, our team and our patients. The idea of separation created by titles and roles is well exampled in the theory of **binary thinking** which demonstrates how we can create our own identities by comparing and contrasting ourself with others (Davies, 2004).

We like to identify ourselves in various different ways as perhaps a parent, a partner, a nurse or a student. While these identities mean that we can explain who we are and what we do, they can also create a sense of difference between us and other people.

Exploring the notion of binary identity and how this might apply in the clinical setting may help us to understand some of the ways in which conflict might arise. Within binary logic, 'A' is 'A' and anything that is not 'A' is 'something else'. Translated into the nursing workplace this may be seen as operating as: 'I am a nurse, you are not'; 'I know what is happening here, you do not'; 'I am the powerful professional, you are the compliant patient'; 'I know best, you do not'. You may have experienced this type of feeling yourself perhaps as a student nurse, or in relation to another more 'powerful' professional.

In part, the differences expressed here represent some of the more negative aspects of creating for ourselves a professional identity which excludes others who do not share our identity (as a nurse, say) – sometimes called **'othering'**. This way of looking at ourselves creates a scheme whereby we see patients and non nursing colleagues as 'other'. It is a small step from seeing ourselves as something different and set apart to the creation of conflict.

Conflict often arises because of perceived, if not real, differences between the needs, wants and desires of individuals. When we as nurses, and nurse leaders, remember that we are people first and nurses second it will allow us to start to see something of the nature of the fear that being 'the other' brings. This realisation will help enable us to not only respond to, but to pre-empt, some of the conflict that arises as a result of fear and perceived isolation.

Activity 4.2 *Critical thinking*

Think about what binary thinking says about professional image and presentation of self to others in the care setting. How is binary identity used in the care setting to advantage the professional? Can you think of times someone has made you feel different or excluded by their behaviour? Have you used binary thinking to your own advantage? What approaches to self presentation and leadership can stop these sorts of situations arising?

There are some possible answers and thoughts at the end of the chapter.

It is worth thinking critically about this example here, not because it is a clever way of understanding how we create identities but because it reflects a way in which conflict may be generated. Quite clearly from this theory we can see divisions between individuals are readily created when we start to see ourselves as something other than fellow human beings. This idea translates well into how we might think about preventing conflict as well as how we lead others by example in the ways in which we interact with our managers, peers, those who work under our leadership and our patients.

Conflict may also arise in the clinical setting when staff disagree about the care and management of a particular patient. Sometimes conflict may arise because of some ethical dilemma such as a family requesting that a loved one is not told their diagnosis when it appears they should be. When ethical dilemmas occur, they can give rise to conflict between people with different views about how the issue should be resolved. Differences of views may then arise along professional boundaries, or between professionals and patients. Alternatively, they may result as a consequence of age, gender, status, culture, religion or experience (Northam, 2009a).

Binary theory helps us to understand what is going on in such situations where conflict arises. People who disagree with our point of view instead of being accepted as people with another viewpoint are regarded as 'other' and therefore become a legitimate target of attack. The role of the leader or manager in such situations is to focus the discussions back to the issue under dispute and away from the personalities involved.

The Chartered Institute of Personnel and Development (2007) identified general behaviour, disputes about performance, attendance at work and relationships between colleagues as being the main causes of conflict at work. Of note, people in public sector employment rated relationships, bullying and harassment and all forms of discriminatory behaviour as being among the major causes of conflict at work.

Bullying takes many forms in the healthcare sector and can involve staff bullying other staff, staff bullying patients, patients bullying staff and visitors and relatives bullying staff. In a survey of NHS staff, 10 per cent reported having been bullied, harassed or abused in the last year by other NHS staff (NHS Employers, 2006).

Bullying can take many forms. Some bullying is deliberate, while other bullying arises out of differences in perception and poor communication. Gossiping about someone, spreading rumours, ridiculing someone as well as being consistently rude or abusive, all constitute bullying behaviour.

Case study: Bullying

Steve was a newly qualified nurse who prior to becoming a nurse had undertaken a first degree and Master's degree in biology. Steve joined the team in the intensive care unit at his local hospital as a junior staff nurse and greatly enjoyed his job.

Amanda was one of the unit sisters who had been qualified for many years and was a very experienced nurse. When Steve was on shift with Amanda he was often allocated the patient in the isolation room. Steve got the feeling that Amanda did not like him and noticed that he was often overlooked for breaks and was never allowed to look after unusual cases in the main unit when she was on duty.

continued opposite...

continued...

Steve felt that he was being bullied and started to become very unhappy at work. Steve raised his concerns with one of the unit charge nurses, Des. Des had also noticed the behaviours that Steve described and advised Steve to have a word with Amanda about it. When Steve asked to talk to Amanda, she was dismissive but Steve persisted. In the office Steve raised his concerns, saying he had joined the team to learn how to nurse in ITU and he was keen to be useful. He said he felt excluded by Amanda and that she appeared to have taken a dislike to him for no apparent reason. Amanda started to cry.

Amanda admitted that she too felt intimidated by Steve as she had found out he had two degrees and she did not even have a diploma. Amanda admitted she was worried about her position in the team with bright young things threatening her status.

In this real life case study, we can see that Amanda's behaviour has arisen out of her own fears about her position in the team. It could have all been so different however; she might have treated Steve in the manner she did because she did not like men, he was gay, from a different ethnic background or she did not like his religious views. Quite clearly any one of these alternative explanations is unacceptable, as is the fact that she was using her position to bully him because she felt threatened.

Activity 4.3	*Evidence-based practice and research*

Unfortunately, bullying and harassment are common workplace occurrences (see the statistics cited earlier). When you are next at work, find a copy of the local bullying and harassment policy and familiarise yourself with the definitions it contains as well as the local practices in relation to it. You may want to repeat this exercise when you are in university: you may find these policies on the local intranet.

As the answers to this activity will depend on the policy available in your own workplace, no outline answer is given.

What all of the examples of how conflict could emerge in the clinical setting have in common is that they all come about as a result of communication issues. Handling communication, perception and relationships is therefore an important element of conflict management.

Managing to reduce the potential for conflict

What we have seen so far in this chapter points to the fact that much conflict can be avoided. From the leadership and management perspective, as well as from the perspective of individual behaviours, there are a number of strategies which can be used to help prevent conflict. The key to reducing the potential for conflict lies in managing the environment of care in such a way that it is focused on achieving high quality patient outcomes. Hocking (2006, page 250) suggests that the route to achieving this is 'through open communication, trust, and accountability'.

There is good reason to think as a leader or manager that treating the staff in our team as people first and as staff second can lead to an increase in the level of trust and reduce the potential for conflict. When team members trust a leader, they are more likely to work co-operatively and less likely to act negatively towards each other and those around them, creating less opportunity for conflict to arise (Kramer, Brewer and Hanna, 1995).

The strategies for managing to reduce the potential for conflict are, like so many issues and ideas in leadership and management, heavily interlinked. The culture of the organisation, department or team all contribute to the ways in which conflict arises, is prevented, recognised and dealt with. Creating a culture where we learn from our mistakes and create environments which allow people to develop and grow as individuals and professionals will have a great impact on the likelihood of conflict arising in a team. While **learning organisations** are explored in more depth in Chapter 8, it is worth noting here that an organisation which allows people to make mistakes, learn from their mistakes and develop is more likely to minimise the likelihood of conflict arising and to handle conflict in a meaningful way. The same message translates well down to team level where a manager that encourages and supports learning enables members of the team to understand the root causes of conflict and how to deal with them.

Managing situations where conflict arises

When conflict does arise, there are a number of approaches that can be taken to manage it. The choice of which approaches to use will depend on the nature of the conflict: who is involved, where it is taking place and whether the conflict is physical or purely verbal in nature. The choice of approach to managing the situation will make a great deal of difference to the potential outcome of the situation. Thought should always be given to what strategy is right to employ in any given situation, but if this is not possible it is always best to start with the minimum intervention required and scale up.

The following table gives some ideas about general approaches to managing conflict, along with when to use them and their pros and cons.

Collaboration: creates a potential situation where everyone can win and allows for creative solutions. It requires that the situation is worked through and a solution found which addresses concerns. This is useful where the conflict arises between individuals who either trust each other a lot or where there is pre-existing enmity. Collaboration, while it may be an effective means of managing conflict, can be time consuming and is open to abuse if both parties are not really committed to it.

Compromising: leads to a situation where everyone involved has to give a little ground. This may prove beneficial where the parties in the dispute are equally committed to their own point of view and where they are of similar status. It can speed up the process of resolving a dispute, but only when the exact outcome is not too important. Compromise may lead to a solution that is not acceptable to anyone and may not work if the sides are too far apart at the start.

— continued opposite...

continued...

Accommodating: is useful when one side of a conflict realises the issue is more important to the other side, or that they are wrong. Accommodating now allows for **social capital** to be built up and called upon later and helps maintain relationships which may be more important than the disagreement. The problem with being accommodating is that people may see it as a sign of weakness and take advantage.

Competing: sometimes other avenues of reaching agreement have been worn out so when the point being made is correct it is important not to give in easily. On other occasions when someone is trying to forcibly get their way it is best to challenge them. The experienced leader or manager will recognise that competition can escalate some conflicts and it may not be wise when the conflict is or may become physical in nature.

Dodging: is perhaps the best strategy when the conflict is not important, you are too busy to deal with an issue at that time, you need to cool off or there is no chance of winning. Dodging the issue can, however, make matters worse in the long run and may allow a transgressor to win. Dodging can be used as a short-term strategy by the manager but rarely results in a satisfactory solution to issue of conflict.

Table 4.1 General approaches to managing conflict situations

Source: Adapted from Thomas and Kilmann (1974)

What seems clear from the strategies above is that different approaches will suit different scenarios. Constant use of one strategy will lead people to thinking that you do not have the **emotional intelligence** to work out when to change what you do in response to different situations. Knowing what strategy to employ is not something that is easily taught and, like emotional intelligence, it is something that comes with time, experience and reflection.

Activity 4.4   *Critical thinking*

Sue has been admitted to the orthopaedic ward following a fall in which she broke her arm. It is late evening and just as visiting is about to finish Dave, Sue's husband, arrives to visit her. You are asked by the ward sister to tell Dave that he must leave in five minutes, despite him having just arrived. Dutifully you tell Dave that visiting is nearly over and he must leave. Dave is angered by this and aggressively states that he has only just been able to get there and he should be allowed to see his wife and that the rules are ridiculous.

Use the strategies identified in Table 4.1 to think about the alternative approaches you might use to handle this situation. Which approach(es) best fit this particular scenario? Why?

There are some possible answers and thoughts at the end of the chapter.

This activity drawn from a recent real life experience demonstrates how rigid adherence to rules can be construed as insensitivity and so inflames what must already be a worrying situation. Clearly the right approach would have been not to provoke conflict in the first place, but to ask whether Dave knew the visiting times and why he had been so late. Perhaps a compromise might then have been reached without the need for generating bad feeling.

There is a key message for the novice manager that rules are sometimes there more as guidelines to follow than rigid policy. The emotionally intelligent manager will realise that on occasions breaking the rules is the right thing to do and that in exercising wise choices such as this they are demonstrating leadership rather than being weak.

Negotiation

Although it is easy to imagine **negotiation** is the starting point for dealing with all conflicts, in some instances it is not. Negotiation means trying to reach an agreement with another party when both parties share the same overall objective but perhaps differ on how this objective might be achieved. Negotiating is the process that is undertaken in order to reach a compromise solution to an issue. One of the fringe benefits of successful negotiation is that the relationship that builds up in a successful negotiation may lead to future collaboration.

The first rule of negotiation is to know what it is you want to achieve – the outcome that is acceptable to you. Once you know what is acceptable as a solution you know what ground you can give in the process and what you need to defend to achieve your goal. This is also the time to decide what the points of conflict are: why do you and the other party not agree?

The second most important negotiating skill is listening (Northam, 2009b). Listening not only allows you to understand the other person's point of view, it also creates opportunity for you to ask sensible questions about what they are saying.

The third rule of negotiation is to build on small successes, get agreement on small issues and then work up towards the main issue of the conflict. This allows for an environment of collaboration and agreement to be created and built upon. What are you willing to give up, and what is the other party willing to give up as part of the process?

Activity 4.5   *Reflection*

Think back to some occasion when you have had a disagreement with someone. A good example might be in the classroom when you have debated the rights and wrongs of the care of a patient with your fellow students. What skills did you use to make your case? Did you listen to what the other side was saying? How did you reach a conclusion?

There are some possible answers and thoughts at the end of the chapter.

Mediation

Sometimes a dispute or conflict between individuals cannot be resolved by the individuals themselves. At this stage there is a need for a third party to help find a resolution to the issue. One approach to conflict resolution is the use of **mediation**. Mediation is not about the settlement of a dispute by the imposition of an agreement; rather it is a means of facilitating a resolution that both parties can agree to. A mediator's role is that of an impartial third party who helps progress a solution to a problem.

In mediation, the mediator listens to both sides of an issue, sometimes in private, and then brings the two sides together to discuss their grievances. The mediator will try to identify common ground, things the two parties can agree on, and uses these in order to start building a resolution to a problem. Fundamental to the process of mediation is that both sides in a dispute agree to take part in the mediation process and that they are both willing to seek agreement. Reaching agreement is not simply about compromise, or one side backing down; instead mediation seeks to build on small agreements until a consensus is reached.

Mediation is especially useful where two sides have a history of not working together as it helps to build relationships which allow for future development and joint working. For a leader, this may mean facilitating discussions between two members of a team who do not get on or who are in conflict about some aspect of their working life.

Arbitration

When the processes of negotiation or mediation fail, it may become necessary to look for other ways of resolving a dispute between two parties. Arbitration and conciliation, like mediation, employ the services of a third, impartial, individual to help reach a resolution.

In arbitration, the role of the third party is to decide on and impose a final solution to the conflict. The decision that is reached is based on the third party gathering together all of the facts and coming to some conclusion about what should be done to resolve the issue. An arbitrator has the authority to impose the decision on those in dispute – however, there may be instances when one, or both, sides in a dispute feel unhappy about the result, creating continued tensions in the workplace. Leaders who have to arbitrate will therefore need to stick to their values and demonstrate emotional intelligence in managing such situations.

Case study: The rota

Ann and Claire are junior staff nurses on the same ward. There is a concert by a well known band in the town in a couple of weekends' time and both Ann and Claire want to go. Both nurses are rostered to be at work at the time of the concert and so both approach the ward sister and ask for an early shift or the day off instead. The sister says that she needs one of them to work and that they must sort it out between them.

Ann and Claire, who aren't the best of friends anyway, soon get into a verbal fight about who should have the opportunity to go to the concert. The argument spills over from the staff room to the ward and the sister has to take them both into her office. Both Ann and Claire claim they need to have the evening off the most and again begin to squabble. The sister has to intervene and suggests that she will have to make the decision and they will have to abide by it as that is what is required. Reluctantly they both agree. The sister says that, as she cannot choose between them, then the original rota which was written without any knowledge of the concert must stand.

Whistle blowing

So far, the examples we have used all have some reasonable explanation and resolving the issues they create is relatively easy. Sadly, this is not always the case. Sometimes there are situations of conflict, bullying or harassment which are not amenable to being dealt with locally. **Whistle blowing** offers one avenue for people who witness, or who are experiencing, conflict or bullying in the workplace to get help.

Essentially, whistle blowing is the act of bringing an important issue to the attention of someone in authority. Sometimes whistle blowing occurs within a team or organisation. If there are issues with an organisation, however, whistle blowing may need to be external. Within the NHS there are policies in place for both forms of whistle blowing. In certain circumstances, these allow the whistle blower to remain anonymous.

The Public Information Disclosures Act 1998 protects people who blow the whistle about poor practices specifically where the worker has real concerns about any one of a number of issues (www.legislation.gov.uk/ukpga/1998/23/contents). Such issues for the manager or leader may include the health and safety of workers. As discussed earlier, this includes protecting staff from abuse and conflict and the subsequent impact of this on their health.

Activity 4.6	*Evidence-based practice and research*

When you are next at work find a copy of the local whistle blowing policy and familiarise yourself with what it says. You may want to repeat this exercise when you are in university: you may find these policies on the local intranet.

As the answers to this activity will depend on the policy available in your own workplace, no outline answer is given.

Deciding to blow the whistle is a big step for anyone involved in conflict or bullying. In all such situations it is better if possible to try to come to some solution more locally. However, there are times, perhaps involving a legal or ethical issue, where whistle blowing may be the right thing to do.

Managing yourself

It may seem strange to say this towards the end of a chapter of dealing with conflict, but the first point of reference for anyone involved in conflict is to ask if they are, themself, the problem. Management of yourself and your relationships with other people is an important step on the road to becoming an effective leader and manager of others. Who wants to be led by someone who cannot manage themself?

Since differences of opinion, perception and power all play a role in creating conflict situations, it is important for a prospective leader and manager to be aware of the influences on their thinking as well as how they come across to others. It may be tempting to think that this can be achieved purely through reflection, but reflection alone is likely to produce a flawed view. Self management is as much about self development as it is about being aware of your own opinions, and if you are to develop you need to take on board feedback from other individuals.

It would be easy to say that in order to avoid unnecessary conflict you should always follow what you believe to be the moral and ethical thing to do. This oversimplifies the case for self management however. Evidently there are some ethical and moral principles which, if you believe in them and act on them, will mean you can usually justify your actions. Such principles might include treating others as equals and always trying to be fair. Rigid adherence to rules, as we saw in Activity 4.4, can lead to problems and so part of managing yourself is to learn when to adapt what you do to the situation. This means being open to the views of others and being able to adapt your behaviours when necessary while not abandoning important ethical principles.

In essence this is about good communication, awareness of how others see you and how you behave and being aware of the perception of others. Mayer and Salovey (1993, page 433) termed this ability emotional intelligence and described it as 'a type of social intelligence that involves the ability to monitor one's own and others' emotions, to discriminate among them, and to use the information to guide one's thinking and actions'. There are essentially four elements to the Mayer–Salovey model of emotional intelligence: the ability to identify emotions in yourself and others; the ability to use emotion to communicate; the ability to understand how emotional information is used to construct meaning; and the ability to manage your own emotions.

Being able to read and understand the emotions that lie behind your own behaviours and the behaviours of others is helpful in identifying whether conflict is a result of your behaviours or a reasonable response to the behaviours of others. To grow your emotional intelligence, it is important to reflect on your own motivations; to ask others about their motivations, and to put this in the context of the situation in which you find yourself. The essence of conflict management, therefore, is honest communication with yourself and with others.

Chapter summary

In this chapter we have identified some of the causes of conflict which arise in the clinical setting. We have identified that perception plays a large part in how people feel about a situation and that poor management of a situation, often the result of poor or non-existent communication, is often the root cause of conflict.

We have identified that there are a number of strategies that can be employed by the nurse to prevent conflict from arising; to identify situations in which conflict may arise and to manage conflict when it does occur. The fundamental messages for the management of conflict appear to lie in the need for good communication, management of self and treating others as equals.

We have seen that not all conflict can be dealt with by the individuals involved in the conflict, and that it is sometimes necessary to involve a third party to either help those in conflict come to a negotiated settlement or to have a settlement imposed. As with all aspects of nursing and interpersonal relationships, the key skill of reflection (both alone and with others) is helpful in resolving situations that arise.

Activities: Brief outline answers

Activity 4.1 (page 60)

Entering a new clinical area for the first time may have made you feel quite unsure about yourself and your own abilities and capacity to fit into the team. You may have been uncertain about where everything is kept and what the routine of the area is, as well as what would be expected of you. Some kind staff would tell you not to worry and might perhaps show you where things were and explain what they expected of you, while others might ignore you or make it quite plain that they were not happy about someone who was unable to pull their weight. The people you most admired and who most put you at your ease would probably be the staff who wanted to share their knowledge with you and who reassured you that in time you would understand what was expected of you as well as how to work effectively within the team.

Patients and visitors feel the same emotions. They are worried about what might happen, what is expected of them, who they will meet and how they will be treated. They also have the concerns that accompany being a consumer of healthcare, what the long-term outcomes might be, how they will be treated and who will be caring for them. Unlike the staff they do not have the luxury of going home at the end of the shift nor of having an education and training that prepares them to understand and make sense of their care. Because of this, they may well feel frightened and vulnerable; some may become aggressive or confrontational in order to hide their vulnerability.

Activity 4.2 (page 61)

The answers to this issue lie in the way in which we choose to present ourselves to others, as well as the values we hold and the ways in which we choose to express these values. If we are quite clear in our interactions with patients and more junior staff that we are the knowledgeable professional and they are not, we will cause antagonism. If we choose to remember, as nurses and leaders of people, that we too are people and that we are dealing with people, then the ways in which we interact will demonstrate this and will be less likely to give rise to behaviours that cause conflict to occur.

Activity 4.4 (page 65)

Collaboration: will require a discussion to take place about Dave's concerns and that you show understanding in reaching a solution which addresses them.

Compromising: will allow you to reach a mutually agreeable solution with Dave – perhaps allowing him to stay a little longer, but only on this occasion.

Accommodating: allowing Dave to stay because of the circumstances would perhaps seem reasonable and will defuse the situation, but it may mean he abuses the system in the future.

Competing: would mean demanding Dave leaves and perhaps calling security. This would alienate both Dave and Sue, and may not be a good idea in the long run.

Dodging: just walking away and hoping Dave will leave is not really an option as other patients in the ward will see what has happened and may choose to do the same with their visitors or may be disturbed by Dave's continued presence.

Activity 4.5 (page 66)

In the classroom setting when discussing the care of a patient, there is usually more than one view about what constitutes the best care. This may hinge on ideas such as patient consent, the cost of the care, the usefulness of the care (or not) or what delivering care in a certain way will mean for other people. What is rarely the case is that people in the room disagree about what they are trying to achieve as almost all care professionals want to achieve the best they can for the patient. You will often find in such negotiations, even if they become a little heated, that the conclusions you come to hinge around the exact context of the case that is under discussion. When people have a different perception of the context, they will disagree. Even when they agree on context they might disagree about the exact nature of the care to be given, but will probably agree to disagree.

Further reading

Bach, S and Gilbert, A (2011) *Communication and Interpersonal Skills for Nurses* (2nd edition). Exeter: Learning Matters. See especially Chapter 4 on Understanding potential barriers to safe and effective practice.

Benson, G, Ploeg, J and Brown, B (2010) A Cross-sectional Study of Emotional Intelligence in Baccalaureate Nursing Students. *Nurse Education Today*, 30 (1): 49–53.
A study of emotional intelligence in nursing students and how it changes across the years of training.

Hocking, BA (2006) Using Reflection to Resolve Conflict. *Journal of the Association of Operating Room Nurses*, 84 (2): 249–59.
A helpful view of conflict management.

Thomas, J (2006) *Survival Guide for Ward Managers, Sisters and Charge Nurses*. London: Churchill Livingstone, Elsevier.
See especially the chapter on dealing with complaints.

Wedderburn Tate, C (2006) The Art of Managing Difficult People. *Nursing Standard*, 20 (19): 72.
A brief but interesting look at managing difficult people.

Useful websites

**www.cipd.co.uk/NR/rdonlyres/1EB2AE66-D1A8-4641-AB8B-B6C67D38E6D9/0/
4334ManagingconflictWEB.pdf**
From the Chartered Institute of Personnel and Development, an easily understood guide to managing conflict at the personal and team level.

www.acas.org.uk/CHttpHandler.ashx?id=960&p=0
The Advisory, Conciliation and Arbitration Service's guide to managing conflict at work.

www.nmc-uk.org/Nurses-and-midwives/Raising-and-escalating-concerns
The nursing and midwifery council's guidance on raising concerns and whistle blowing.

www.pcaw.co.uk
Public Concern at Work is the independent charitable authority on public interest whistle blowing.

**www.dh.gov.uk/en/Publicationsandstatistics/Publications/
PublicationsPolicyAndGuidance/DH_4050929**
NHS whistle blowing guidance.

www.bristol-inquiry.org.uk/index.htm
The Bristol Inquiry into children's heart surgery and related deaths. Includes statements from whistle blowers.

www.cipd.co.uk/subjects/lrnanddev/selfdev/emotintel.htm?IsSrchRes=1
The Chartered Institute of Personnel and Development's accessible guide to emotional intelligence.

Chapter 5
Coaching, mentoring and clinical supervision

NMC Standards for Pre-registration Nursing Education

This chapter will address the following competencies:

Domain 2: Communication and interpersonal skills

1. All nurses must build partnerships and therapeutic relationships through safe, effective and non-discriminatory communication. They must take account of individual differences, capabilities and needs.

Domain 4: Leadership, management and team working

4. All nurses must be self-aware and recognise how their own values, principles and assumptions may affect their practice. They must maintain their own personal and professional development, learning from experience, through supervision, feedback, reflection and evaluation.

5. All nurses must facilitate nursing students and others to develop their competence, using a range of professional and personal development skills.

Essential Skills Clusters

This chapter will address the following ESCs:

Cluster: Organisational aspects of care

12. People can trust the newly registered graduate nurse to respond to their feedback and a wide range of other sources to learn, develop and improve services.

14. People can trust the newly registered graduate nurse to be an autonomous and confident member of the multi-disciplinary or multi agency team and to inspire confidence in others.

17. People can trust the newly registered graduate nurse to work safely under pressure and maintain the safety of service users at all times.

Chapter aims

After reading this chapter, you will be able to:

- identify different coaching methods;
- recognise diverse mentoring roles and how they can be used effectively;

continued opposite...

continued...

- understand the benefits of clinical supervision;
- recognise the signs of burnout and methods to reduce these effects.

Introduction

The main emphasis in this chapter is on the support of staff through leadership and management techniques such as coaching, mentoring and clinical supervision. This chapter will investigate when to coach to improve performance or achievements. Different forms of coaching and mentoring, whether in an educational role or as a supporting role model, will be discussed and compared as methods of staff support. Problem solving and decision making frameworks are included in the discussion on coaching techniques. Clinical supervision models will also be introduced and discussed. The concept of a learning culture will be explored. The detrimental effects of staff burnout will be considered here as will the notion of establishing a workplace environment that embraces the philosophy of work-life balance.

Coaching to improve performance

The term 'coaching' is more often used in the UK when referring to the training of athletes or performers, and may be caricatured by a person with a whistle and clipboard.

Increasingly the term refers to an approach to encouraging the improved performance of skills based upon an interpersonal relationship between a manager or team leader and a team member. In Chapter 3, we spoke about staff development and touched on performance appraisal as a means of planning and supporting staff to improve their knowledge and skills. Coaching is one method of supporting others to improve in an individually tailored manner. It is based upon a belief that individuals can develop skills and knowledge through frequent interactions (often called one-to-one meetings or 1:1s) that are planned and carried out with an agreed outcome in mind.

The notion of coaching in organisations, and mentoring which we will look at later in the chapter, as a management tool began with the introduction of the people management and development literature. It can be traced back to the situational leadership model developed by Hersey and Blanchard in the 1960s (Hersey, Blanchard and Johnson, 2007). The model is composed of four quadrants (Figure 5.1). Hersey and Blanchard's use of the term coaching is meant to convey leading and persuading to adopt a solution to the situation. In this way the member of staff is included in the decision making and involved in suggestions for completing the task. It is an approach that encourages motivation as well as building competence.

In Chapter 3 (Working with individuals in teams) we explored the work of Kotter (1990), who recognised the importance of matching the approach with the characteristics of the individual. He developed a scheme for matching the appropriate leadership style to an individual's levels of

Figure 5.1: Adapted from Hersey and Blanchard's Situational Leadership Model

Source: Adapted from Hersey et al. (2007)

commitment and competence to identify when and how tasks should be delegated. This enables a leader to draw out the best in their team members and identify where development needs to take place. The Hersey and Blanchard model extends this approach and stresses that the leader has to be flexible and have at the forefront the developmental needs of the individual and not only the appropriate delegation method.

The leader needs to select an approach, or combination of approaches, from one of four leadership styles:

- telling/directing;
- selling/coaching;
- participating/supporting;
- delegating.

These are matched with one of four follower styles, or developmental level of maturity in the individual:

- high competence/high commitment;
- high competence/variable commitment;
- some competence/low commitment;
- low competence/high commitment.

Depending on the maturational level of the person the leader provides high to low support along an axis of low to high direction. For example, the person with high commitment/high competence requires the least support and direction and can assume delegated tasks with minimal interference from the leader.

Case study: Teaching a procedure

David is a grade 6 staff nurse, and Jasmine a new healthcare assistant. On Jasmine's second day, David spends 30 minutes telling her how to carry out a procedure to clean and redress a wound with the expectation that she will to do this herself once the knowledge and skills required for the task have been thoroughly explained. David gives Jasmine instructions on what to use, why, when, where and to whom. Then he tells her he will come back in two hours' time to see how she is getting on.

When David returns, the wound has not been dressed with the appropriate dressing and he has to redo the dressing. This causes unnecessary discomfort to the patient and wastes time.

Although David may feel frustrated about this, questions have to be asked about the process of instruction that took place and whether it can be improved. Hersey and Blanchard would say that leaders have to match the style of leadership to the maturity (or developmental style) and readiness (i.e. their competence and motivation) of the person or team they are leading to perform a task. Thus, a simple telling and instruction session will not be sufficient. There needs to be an assessment of the individual's learning style, level of comprehension, confidence, motivation and a relationship established or developed between the leader and the 'follower'.

This means that David, as the senior, might be advised to take the following steps:

1. *Make an overall assessment of Jasmine's scope of current tasks and activities. Determine her current workload and how she is coping with it.*
2. *Assess Jasmine's development level on the requested task by questioning and/or demonstration.*
3. *Decide on the leadership style.*
4. *Discuss with Jasmine the approach to be taken.*
5. *Follow up and discuss progress, correct where necessary.*

Activity 5.1 *Reflection*

Reading the case study above, imagine that you are the leader of the team on a shift in a busy female medical ward and are asking a junior member of staff to undertake a task similar to the one delegated to Jasmine in the scenario. Write out an imaginary short story of how you would have tackled the five steps above. What factors would you take into account? You may want to revise your knowledge of Mumford's (1999) learning styles to help you consider how individuals learn. A web link is in the useful websites section at the end of the chapter to help you here. Which leadership approach would you take to coach the junior member of staff based upon your version of events? Try to see it from the junior staff's point of view as well as the senior's perspective.

As this answer is based on your own reflection, there is no outline answer at the end of the chapter.

Since the introduction of situational leadership other approaches have been developed in coaching methods for work improvement. In the UK, the notion of coaching as a metaphor for improving performance came to prominence with the publication of *The Inner Game of Tennis*

(1974) by Tim Gallway, who went on to publish *The Inner Game of Work* (2000). The latter drew on a philosophy summarised as *'Performance = Potential minus Interference'*. Thus the coach's job was to release the self knowledge and potential that everyone possesses rather than deliberately instructing an individual towards achievements. The key ingredient was to develop greater self-awareness and a sense of responsibility in the performer. Since these early proposals, and a call for more evidence-based approaches utilising such philosophies, a body of literature has grown to support the coaching approach (Grant, 2001).

The GROW technique

Developed from the original Gallway texts is a coaching technique that relies on using questions and which follows a structure to involve the person in problem solving as well as learning. Known as the 'GROW' technique, the idea is to use a simple guided set of questions that can form the basis of a discussion in a coaching session or as a means to establishing the developmental level of a person to be supported. The aim is to assist the person to think about the problem/task at hand and identify a solution or range of options.

An easy way to remember the structure of the questions is to refer to the mnemonic that summarises the GROW technique in this way:

- establish the **G**oal;
- examine the **R**eality;
- consider all **O**ptions;
- confirm the **W**ill to act.

This approach has been found to be helpful in improving motivation with a person who has basic knowledge, expertise and enthusiasm. However, with inexperienced learners this can be time consuming and not practical for day-to-day work-based situations (Parsloe and Leedham, 2009). For this approach to be effective the questions need to be expanded, undertaken over a period of time and yet remain focused on the main goal to be achieved. The prominent factor is that the coaching is undertaken as a conversation with two-way communication between the person and the leader or manager.

The 3 D technique

A more rapid approach is known as the 3 D technique. When time is really short and a solution to a problem has to be identified quickly the technique is to identify elements on three dimensions:

1. The situation – for example timescales, lack of resources, lack of expertise.
2. People involved – for example unhappy, impatient, unreliable, over confident.
3. You – lack of knowledge, conflicting priorities, general attitude.

From this analysis it is possible, by using questioning techniques around the dimensions, to draw out potential actions or plans.

Activity 5.2	*Reflection*

This activity is designed to help you with rapid coaching skill building.

Practice the 3 D technique on yourself to coach yourself through a problem by following the following steps:

1. Define a current problem in a single sentence.
2. List three general issues relating to the problem situation.
3. List three issues relating to the people involved.
4. List three issues that relate specifically to you and the problem.
5. Choose one issue from each of your three lists of three issues.
6. Now identify one or more actions/options that are most likely to make progress in solving the problem.

As you are going through the steps, imagine you are asking yourself questions and make a note of the coaching questions you ask, to reflect later if they were the right questions to ask.

You may want to gain further skills in this approach by working with a fellow student or friend on a problem either you or they wish to solve. In this way you not only develop your own skills, you can also ask for feedback on the different types of questions you need to ask to elicit answers that are helpful from your colleague or friend.

As this answer is based on your own reflection, there is no outline answer at the end of the chapter.

You may now be thinking that there is an overlap between the role of coach and the mentorship role you are experiencing in your practice learning and you would be right. However, there are subtle differences which we will look at in the next section.

Mentoring

Mentor was the name of a character in Greek mythology, the tutor of Odysseus' son Telemachus in Homer's *Odyssey*. So he could hardly be more different from the person with a whistle and clipboard described on page 73.

The tutoring Mentor offered was not restricted to the giving of information; rather he encouraged the exploration of such subjects as virtue, integrity, responsibility and character development. He was a trusted and wise counsellor. This historical meaning has remained in use over time and is still used today for someone who has acted as a role model or who has had a significant influence on a person's career or professional outlook on life. The term 'coach' is a more recent one and is used specifically to describe the transport of skills and knowledge towards a higher or improved level.

Confusingly, coaching can also be incorporated into a mentoring role. The term mentoring, today, can cover several roles such as coach, adviser, guide, confidant/e, teacher, role model, counsellor, friend, consultant, critic and advocate. The NMC has identified standards for mentors of nursing and midwifery students. There is no definition of mentoring in the NMC standards; however, there are criteria that have to be met to support learning and assessing of students in practice.

Activity 5.3   *Evidence-based practice and research*

Go to the website address in the useful websites section for the NMC Standards to Support Learning and Assessing in Practice and review the standards in Section 2 for mentoring. Think about how you will undertake this role when you become a qualified nurse and how you will plan to take a recognised mentorship education programme.

This activity aims to help you understand more fully the role of mentoring nursing students but also encourages you to think about your own personal development plan as well as your engagement with the notion of lifelong learning.

You may want to discuss with your mentor their experience of taking the mentoring course and their experience of being a mentor to students. Reflect on what you can learn from their experiences.

As a final part of this research activity, ask your mentor if they had or have a mentor now that they are qualified and, if they have, what impact this has had on their working lives.

As this answer is based on your own research and reflections, there is no outline answer at the end of the chapter.

Research summary: Multi-professional views of mentorship

Bray and Nettleton (2007) researched the role of the mentor in nursing, midwifery and medicine using questionnaires and semi structured telephone interviews with both mentors and mentees. They were interested in any differences in the professional perceptions of the role. They were also interested in the potential dilemma that mentors, who are perceived as wise guides, have to become assessors and make judgements on their mentees' abilities. This could be viewed as a conflict of interest. They found that for nurse mentors the roles of teacher, supporter and role model were most important with only 5 per cent indicating assessor as part of the role. By contrast, in midwifery the role of facilitator came higher than teacher and similarly few regarding assessor as part of the role. Within medicine, advisor and supporter were regarded as most important with only 2 per cent regarding assessing as important.

When asked about any aspect of the role they found most difficult both nurses and midwives reported difficulties in being objective towards their students when they had become 'supportive friends'. In medicine, less difficulty was reported with the assessor role. The biggest difficulty was finding time to commit to the role and all its aspects.

Bray and Nettleton found that across the professions there was a lack of clarity about the combination of a role of assessor with mentor. They admit that they had a small sample and have reservations about the generalisability of their findings. Yet,

continued opposite...

continued...

they make an interesting observation that as we move towards further collaboration within multi-disciplinary professional teams a multi-professional approach should be adopted towards defining the role and function of mentoring in healthcare professional education.

Mentoring in other contexts

While we may be familiar with mentoring in healthcare settings, it is worth noting that mentoring takes place in other sectors and organisations outside of healthcare education. We can learn from these relationships as they provide a contrast to the mentoring experienced in healthcare as well as ideas for opportunities for service development and relationships. This could be to develop entrepreneurial or business skills (see also Chapter 7), or alternatively to enhance working in community settings or with third sector or voluntary services groups in the fields of mental health and learning disabilities. One example can be in business to business relationships where a mentor from a large organisation may work with a small organisation to advise on economic regeneration. In business to social enterprise relationships, organisations like the Princes' Youth Business Trust have mentors to guide young starters who have received grants from the Trust. Similar to this are training schemes supported by the Government.

Providing mentoring to special needs or community projects has become an important part of community university engagement schemes where more personal or individually tailored mentors are matched to individuals (Schuetze and Inman, 2010). Working the other way around, business people can work with education (e.g. head teachers, universities and students) to advise on business skills. There are also buddying schemes between first and third year students, which are another version of mentoring.

Broadly speaking there are three main types:

1. The corporate mentor who is a guide or counsellor in someone's career from orientation into the company to senior management.
2. The qualification mentor who is required by a professional organisation – such as the NMC – to guide candidates towards achieving a qualification. This includes NVQs.
3. The community mentor who acts as a guide or counsellor to individuals who may be disadvantaged, experiencing social inclusion or in a distressing situation (see the Mentoring and Befriending Foundation in the useful websites section at the end of this chapter).

Throughout these discussions there has been a tacit acknowledgement that everyone needs access to guidance or experienced advice at some point in their professional lives. The notion of lifelong learning was mentioned earlier and it is highly relevant in nursing where care may not change but clinical treatments are constantly evolving. Consequently, we need to be prepared to update our practice and ensure that our practice is meeting the needs of the client group with whom we work. Gaining experience in a given field is one way to add to our skills and knowledge. Seeking the guidance of a clinically experienced practitioner is another means to reflect and learn from everyday practice. Often termed clinical supervision, it is the focus of the next section.

Clinical supervision

Thomas (2006) says that some nurses have become too focused on definitions of clinical supervision and that it is simply someone who is more expert than you, with whom you can have regular contact to help reflect and learn (for a more detailed literature review see further reading). She suggests this could be a nurse specialist, a consultant doctor, a nurse consultant or another more experienced ward manager. Thomas maintains that all nurses in a team should have access to clinical supervision. A more junior nurse can be matched to a more experienced nurse who is not a direct assessor or appraiser thus providing a basis for a trusting relationship to develop. The aim is to build up a relationship so that the clinical supervisor can be contacted in times of need, rather than you just meeting them at set times. This model may be suitable for busy acute adult care environments but may not suit all situations, specialties and fields of practice.

Activity 5.4   *Critical thinking*

Supervision can be on a one-to-one basis or in groups. Think about the advantages and disadvantages of each approach and draw up a list to compare.

Further guidance is given on this activity at the end of the chapter.

There are very specific and different statutory requirements for supervision of midwives and the NMC has standards for the selection and activities of supervisors of midwives. In mental health settings, clinical supervision was introduced into pre-registration education in 1994 and in 1995 the United Kingdom Council for Nursing and Midwifery (forerunner of the NMC) declared clinical supervision should be in all fields of nursing and midwifery. The literature suggests the number of nurses receiving clinical supervision varies between regions and specialties. Similarly, the length of time and training for providing supervision is variable.

There do seem to have been technical advances made in the delivery of clinical supervision in community settings using telephone conferencing and similar techniques. However, the majority of research literature concerns the educational provision of clinical supervision in pre-registration nursing courses (Butterworth et al, 2007). Employer organisations and their influence on implementing a culture for clinical supervision are seen as crucial themes in the literature. The factors influencing levels of engagement in organisations appear to be culture, availability of time, supervisor numbers and many local factors. The role of the organisation in creating a culture of learning will be discussed next.

The learning organisation

The concept of the **learning organisation** is seen by many as the way in which organisations will have to organise their structures for the twenty-first century. Up until the mid 1980s it was quite possible to have a successful organisation without mentioning the word *learning*. As we steer ourselves deeply into the territory of the twenty-first century, there is a world of global information and technologically driven organisations. Speed will be important to communicate changes and information management systems become key, which means people and organisations will need to learn to do things differently and quickly. New information is becoming continuously available, requiring new ideas to be adopted and skills and knowledge to be continuously updated.

In healthcare we have seen the implementation in the last ten years of developments such as telemedicine, microsurgery, stem cell research, patient held records, shared patient management systems and many other technological and pharmacological advances. In addition, there are constant pressures to reduce costs and maximise efficiencies which has led to a short-term focus on immediate results and constant efforts to rationalise the number of employees in organisations.

There is a conflict, therefore, between the organisation's need to actively manage the learning potential of its employees and the pressures to change employment practices and professional roles. Not surprisingly, there is a culture of resistance to change if professional status and roles are eroded or services are seen to be reduced.

Case study: Changing the skill mix

The scene is a community healthcare setting. Two new roles have been introduced into the health visiting team to improve the skill mix. Joan, a nursery nurse, is employed to carry out focused parenting skills training over six weeks with families, providing weekly support to learn new skills. Joan is also available for advice at child health clinics. Usha is a staff nurse who used to work on a children's ward. She has a children's nursing qualification and experience, and is now employed to perform three month developmental checks in the home. She is also available for pre-school checks to work with the school nurses. This frees up time for Liz, Jamil and Frances (the three health visitors in the team) to deal with complex family cases and public health initiatives. These kinds of cases have become much more prevalent in their caseloads and while they would like to continue with providing a service to all mothers and their families they realise that they need to focus their specialist expertise on more complicated cases where they can give extra time. Liz, Jamil and Frances are encouraged to undertake specialist, post-qualifying courses in child protection and public health. Joan (the nursery nurse) and Usha (the staff nurse) are also given the opportunity to go on to further training: Joan to become a registered nurse and Usha to become a registered community health visitor and public health nurse. The Team Manager and the organisation (as part of its staff development strategy) is prepared to sponsor them for future training for career development. This also supports the organisation's strategy for succession planning and maintaining a learning culture.

This is an example of where new roles have been introduced into the team that are less costly than the health visitors to employ, which means efficiencies have been made. But Joan and Usha have the potential and ability to make a significant contribution to the work of the team as well as supporting the notion of a learning culture. At the same time the experience and skills of the health visitors, Liz, Jamil and Frances, are maximised and not diminished by the inclusion of new roles into the team.

It is always worth your while looking into the staff development strategy of the organisation you will go to work for after you qualify to see what opportunities there are for you to develop promotion opportunities or a career pathway.

The main features of a learning organisation are:

- An increased focus on learning and development to ensure organisational effectiveness and a sustainable future.
- Encouraging as many people as possible to become coaches, mentors or clinical supervisors to ensure learning takes place in the workplace.
- Establishing training programmes in coaching, mentoring and clinical supervision.
- Generating a culture that accepts the need to move from current standards of performance to higher levels to ensure continuous improvements in performance.
- Supporting individuals to manage their own learning to develop their skills, maximise potential and enable a satisfactory work-life balance (adapted from Parsloe and Leedham, 2009).

Activity 5.5   *Critical thinking*

Parsloe and Leedham (2009) provide strategic level solutions to creating a learning organisation. These are for the senior management teams to consider implementing. Let's think more locally to where you may be working. Imagine you are a new staff nurse on a unit (this could be in a mental health, learning disability, children's hospital or community setting) and you know that several different students have practice experience on the unit – including student nurses, medical students, physiotherapy students, pharmacist students, etc. What practical ideas could you offer in the next team meeting about creating a learning environment and how would you go about this task?

Hints:

1. Would you first find out what kind of students attend the unit and who the mentors are?
2. Would you undertake an informal survey of their views on how to create a learning environment and one that considers, and that would benefit, multi-disciplinary team working if more than one profession is represented?
3. Would you draw on any of your positive learning experiences as a student in other settings?
4. Would you look for any evidence in the literature of other initiatives to create learning environments or evidence to support your initiative?
5. Would you draw up your ideas into a proposal citing the advantages and disadvantages of your ideas and a plan of implementation for discussion in the team meeting?

As this answer is based on your own research and reflections, there is no outline answer at the end of the chapter.

Burnout and work-life balance

Throughout this chapter we have been discussing ways that leaders and managers can support team members and colleagues. With increasingly complex workloads and demanding resource pressures we have to consider the effects this can have on the working life of the individual. In extreme cases many staff experience degrees of burnout. It is important to recognise the early signs of burnout before it takes a hold and also to look at ways to create a work setting that has a philosophy of work-life balance.

Burnout

Burnout is defined as a prolonged response to chronic emotional and interpersonal stressors on the job and is defined by the three overwhelming dimensions of exhaustion, cynicism and sense of inefficacy (Maslach, 2003). Unlike acute stress reactions, which develop in response to specific situations, burnout is a cumulative reaction to work stressors. The emphasis is on the process of gradual psychological erosion and the social outcomes rather than physical outcomes of this chronic exposure. Burnout is therefore the result of prolonged exposure to chronic interpersonal stressors. The predictors are the three dimensions of exhaustion, cynicism and a sense of inefficacy; however, other workplace factors such as working in caregiving environments where a sense of giving with little regard for self, as well as reduced resources, have been found to compound the likelihood of burnout.

Research summary: Burnout

In 2002, as part of a larger survey into the relationship between qualified nursing staff and quality of patient care outcomes, Aiken et al studied the relationship of burnout to qualified nurse/patient ratios. They found that higher emotional exhaustion and increased job dissatisfaction were strongly and significantly associated with nurse/patient ratios. Their findings indicated that increasing a ratio of patients to nurses by one patient could increase emotional exhaustion. This implied that nurses in hospitals with patient ratios of 8:1 nurse would be 2.29 times as likely as nurses with 4:1 ratios to show signs of high emotional exhaustion.

In 2006, Edwards and colleagues surveyed Community Mental Health Nurses using the Maslach Burnout Inventory (MBI) and the Manchester Clinical Supervision Scale (MCSS) to identify whether effective clinical supervision could have a positive effect on burnout. Their findings indicated on the MBI that 36 per cent of staff had high levels of emotional exhaustion, 12 per cent high levels of depersonalisation and 10 per cent had low levels of personal accomplishment. Those nurses who had completed six sessions of clinical supervision scored lower MBI scores and higher scores on the MCSS, which indicated effective supervision (Edwards et al, 2006).

These two studies are examples of the extensive research undertaken in this area and which offer means of early detection and solutions to minimise effects in the workplace.

Work-life balance

Linked to the subject of burnout is the more recent concept of work-life balance. This is about people having a measure of control over when, where and how they work. It is achieved when an individual's right to a fulfilled life inside and outside paid work is accepted and respected as the norm, to the mutual benefit of the individual, business and society. Striking a balance between the needs of the individual employee, customer and organisation demands the following:

- **For employees:** Different individuals will have different expectations and needs at different times in their life.
- **For customers:** Organisations need to respond to the demands of their customers if they are to continue to be successful.
- **For organisations:** Organisations need to be able to manage costs, maintain profitability and ensure that teams work effectively together.

In 2010, an estimated one in five UK workers were mothers; 25 per cent of all families were single parent families, and up to 10 million people were caring for elderly relatives. By 2022 there will be 1 million fewer workers under 50 and 3 million more over 50. We now live in a 'service' world where customers increasingly expect a personalised, 24/7 service (The Work Foundation, 2008). The demands on workers to juggle home life, health and happiness are even greater in the twenty-first century than ever before.

Case study: Work-life balance

This example is from the Good Work Foundation, a not for profit organisation that has the aim to improve working life. The Good Hope Hospital in Birmingham had a project to improve work-life balance through improving recruitment and retention problems. The hospital had 2,841 employees, with 81 per cent women and 14 per cent ethnic minorities. Staff turnover was high at 18 per cent (this includes 12 per cent voluntary leavers but excludes completed contracts such as doctors on six months). Eighty-five per cent of women returned to work after maternity leave.

The NHS in general, including Good Hope Hospital, was facing a recruitment and retention crisis. The response was to introduce a system of self-rostering, whereby nurses choose the shifts they want to work rather than the traditional off-duty system of nurses writing down the shifts they cannot work. The off-duty system, apart from being extremely time consuming, was open to abuse and favouritism and was well recognised as being a cause of friction on wards.

The computerised RosterPro system turned the whole process on its head, and removed the administrative burden from the nurse manager. Once a month nurses simply enter the shifts they want to work onto the computer. As well as identifying their availability, the nurses are able to assign a preference rating to each shift. RosterPro does the rest, with the system allocating shifts on a fair and equitable basis.

Overall benefits were:

- *improved staff morale;*
- *boost in recruitment rates;*
- *reduction in staff turnover from 14.4 per cent to 9.3 per cent;*
- *huge administrative burden released from ward managers;*
- *sickness and absenteeism rates greatly reduced;*

continued opposite...

continued...

- average sickness at *Good Hope* reduced from 6 per cent to 5 per cent (against an increase on wards with no self-rostering);
- better customer care due to staff having a better work-life balance;
- 15 per cent increase in staff being able to work the hours of their choosing in the space of one year;
- improvement in computer literacy amongst nursing staff in practice.

An example of a nurse who has benefited from the introduction of self-rostering is Auveen, a ward sister and mother. Auveen's story can be found on the Work Foundation website, but in short the flexibility of self-rostering allows her to manage her work-life balance so she has time for her husband and children, and her work. Auveen works 37½ hours a week and, using RosterPro, chooses her shifts to allow her to make time for activities with her two young children. For example, if her children have after-school activities or an appointment with the dentist, Auveen can work an early shift to accommodate this. The Work Foundation's account quotes her as saying: 'Whether I'm providing an after-school taxi service or spending time doing homework with the children, I love the fact that my job now allows me this flexibility. I firmly believe that young minds need to be nourished and my working pattern allows me to spend quality time with the children that a fixed hours job just wouldn't allow.'

It may not always be possible to introduce the flexible work scheduling in the example above; however, working creatively with the philosophy of creating a work-life balance in the workplace will go some way to improving difficult working lives. In the useful websites section you will find an A–Z of further ideas which you may wish to take to your workplaces and discuss with your teams.

Chapter summary

In this chapter you have explored three different methods of staff support that can improve staff performance as well as improve work-life balance. Coaching can be used to improve performance and problem solving. It does not have to be undertaken by an expert in the field of practice. Mentoring has many different forms and can include coaching. Clinical supervision is usually undertaken by an expert in the field around a very specific area of knowledge.

It is essential for twenty-first century organisations to create a learning culture if they are to keep abreast of innovations, support staff morale and encourage personal development options. In addition, the pressures of contemporary life need to be supported by initiatives to bring about a balance between work and personal life. Leaders at all levels in the organisation have a part to play in creating these environments.

Activities: Brief outline answers

Activity 5.4 (page 80)

Clinical supervision	Advantages	Disadvantages
Group supervision	• More people seen at one time, saving time • A variety of ideas can be offered from different perspectives • Helps with team building	• Takes more people away from the clinical area at one time • Requires an experienced/trained facilitator • May not meet everyone's specific needs
One-to-one	• More personal and focused • Deeper trusting relationship can be established • Can specifically match specialty advice	• Could become too intense • Personalities may not match • More resources required for time

Further reading

Cummins, A (2009) Clinical Supervision: The Way Forward? A Review of the Literature. *Nurse Education in Practice*, 9: 215–20.
This article gives a more recent review of the clinical supervision literature and how it complements mentorship and preceptorship programmes post qualification.

Parsloe, E and Leedham, M (2009) *Coaching and Mentoring: Practical Conversations to Improve Learning.* London: Kogan Page.
Gives useful detail on how to conduct the coaching conversation and advice on how to deal with difficult conversations.

Thomas, J (2006) *Survival Guide for Ward Managers, Sisters and Charge Nurses.* London: Churchill Livingstone/Elsevier.
A pocket sized, practically focused guide to surviving in a new managerial role. It does what it says in the title and is a very easy quick reference guide.

Useful websites

http://rapidbi.com/created/learningstyles.html#honeymumfordlearningstyleslsq
Learning styles review: several learning styles theories are displayed on this url; however, the overview of Honey and Mumford's four learning styles – activist, reflector, theorist and pragmatist – will be particularly helpful for Activity 5.1.

www.nmc-uk.org/Educators/Standards-for-education/Standards-to-support-learning-and-assessment-in-practice/

Will take you to the *NMC Standards for Nursing and Midwifery Learning*. See Section 2, 2.1 for the standards for mentorship.

www.mandbf.org/projects

Website of the Mentoring and Befriending Foundation.

www.princes-trust.org.uk/?gclid=CNOo467UlqYCFQse4QodWT4kZg

The Prince's Youth Business Trust, which has mentors to guide young starters who have received grants from the Trust.

www.direct.gov.uk/en/Employment/Jobseekers/programmesandservices/DG_180442

Similar to the above are training schemes supported by the Government, as detailed on this site.

www.sayeconomy.com/situational-leadership-by-kenneth-blanchard-and-paul-hersey

The Situational Leadership Model is briefly explained and critiqued on this website, which also shows the full original diagram of the model.

www.theworkfoundation.com/difference/e4wlb/jargonbuster.aspx

The Work Foundation's A–Z of ideas for maintaining work-life balance. The case study from the Good Hope Hospital cited in this chapter can be found at:

www.theworkfoundation.com/Assets/Docs/Publications/GoodHopeHospital.pdf

Chapter 6
Frameworks for management and leadership

NMC Standards for Pre-registration Nursing Education

This chapter will address the following competencies:

Domain 1: Professional values

6. All nurses must understand the roles and responsibilities of other health and social care professionals, and seek to work with them collaboratively for the benefit of all who need care.

Domain 4: Leadership, management and team working

4. All nurses must be self-aware and recognise how their own values, principles and assumptions may affect their practice. They must maintain their own personal and professional development, learning from experience, through supervision, feedback, reflection and evaluation.
6. All nurses must work independently as well as in teams. They must be able to take the lead in co-ordinating, delegating and supervising care safely, managing risk and remaining accountable for the care given.

Essential Skills Clusters

This chapter will address the following ESCs:

Cluster: Organisational aspects of care

14. People can trust the newly registered graduate nurse to be an autonomous and confident member of the multi-disciplinary or multi agency team and to inspire confidence in others.

    At entry to the register:

    7. Challenges the practice of self and others across the multi-professional team.
    8. Takes effective role within the team adopting the leadership role when appropriate.
    9. Act as an effective role model in decision making, taking action and supporting others.

15. People can trust the newly registered graduate nurse to safely delegate to others and to respond appropriately when a task is delegated to them.

    At entry to the register:

    4. Prepares, supports and supervises those to whom care has been delegated.

continued opposite...

continued...

16. People can trust the newly registered graduate nurse to safely lead, co-ordinate and manage care.

At entry to the register:

1. Inspires confidence and provides clear direction to others.
2. Takes decisions and is able to answer for these decisions when required.
4. Acts as a positive role model for others.

Chapter aims

After reading this chapter, you will be able to:

* identify the features of leadership and management;
* discuss what features of management and leadership are appropriate in nursing;
* relate some management and leadership theories to your own experiences of practice;
* consider which aspects of leadership and management you would like to develop in yourself.

Introduction

The purpose of this chapter is to lay bare some of the key definitions and understandings of what it means to be a leader or manager in the health and social care sector. To fully appreciate leadership and management for nursing it is important that any definition of the roles that leaders and managers hold includes not just a theoretical explanation of what they do, but also some explanation of why they are important to practice.

This chapter will advance some of the ideas seen in Chapter 1, where the key characteristics of leaders and managers as might be experienced by student nurses were explored.

Are leadership and management different?

Some commentators on leadership and management regard them to be mutually exclusive ideas; that is, a manager is a manager and a leader is a leader. More commonly, and in our view more correctly, it is perhaps true to say that leadership is one of the roles of a manager in health and social care, whereas leadership can be everyone's responsibility depending on their position, the roles they are given and the situations in which they find themselves.

This may seem a difficult idea to grasp; but consider all the people who display leadership qualities, or who undertake leadership roles, in the clinical setting. These people may include individuals who have responsibility for leading a small team, some of whom may be at the same grade. Other leaders may have specific roles in the team, such as a wound care or lifting and handling co-ordinator. On occasions people may have to show leadership because of a situation that arises. Such individuals are not perhaps always managers, but they are leaders.

Managers on the other hand are most often defined by their position and job title e.g.) a ward manager, community team manager or outpatients manager. While such individuals are managers, part of their role will include displaying some of the activities of leadership as described later in the chapter.

Pascale (1990, page 65) suggests that: 'Managers do things right, while leaders do the right thing.' The suggestion here is that managers are bound by and follow local policy and procedures, while leaders follow their intuition and understanding of people to get things done. In 1989, Bennis famously explored the comparisons between what he saw as the key features of leadership and management. He listed 12 key differences between managers and leaders:

1. Managers administer; Leaders innovate.
2. The Manager is a copy; The Leader is an original.
3. Managers maintain; Leaders develop.
4. Managers focus on systems and structure; Leaders focus on people.
5. Managers rely on control; Leaders inspire trust.
6. Managers have a short-range view; Leaders have a long-range perspective.
7. Managers ask how and when; Leaders ask what and why.
8. Managers have their eye always on the bottom line; the Leader's eye is on the horizon.
9. Managers imitate; Leaders originate.
10. Managers accept the status quo; Leaders challenge it.
11. Managers are the classic good soldier; Leaders are their own person.
12. Managers do things right; Leaders do the right thing.

We can see in these comparisons that managers are regarded as having the interests of the organisation at heart and that they achieve this by following the rules and maintaining the status quo.

Daft (2001) further expands on Bennis' ideas:

13. Managers plan and budget; Leaders create vision and set direction.
14. Managers generally direct and control; Leaders allow room for others to grow, and change them in the process.
15. Managers create boundaries; Leaders reduce them.
16. The Manager's relationship with people is based on position power; the Leader's relationship and influence is based on personal power.
17. Managers act as boss; Leaders act as coaches, facilitators and servants.
18. Managers exhibit and focus on: emotional distance, expert mind, talking, conformity and insight into the organisation; Leaders exhibit and focus on: emotional connectedness, open mindedness, listening, nonconformity and insight into self.
19. Managers maintain stability; Leaders create change.
20. Managers create a culture of efficiency; Leaders create a culture of integrity.

What we can see in these definitions is the focus on emotional connections with the team on the part of the leader, and remoteness and a controlling attitude from the manager. What seems clear from these distinctions is that some of these qualities will suit some situations at different times, but it is unlikely that one or the other approach will always be the right way to deal with all situations that arise in nursing.

It is worth noting here that leadership is also one of the roles of the manager and so the distinctions drawn here may be somewhat artificial. Clearly within the care setting there is a need for nurses to demonstrate the qualities of both leaders and managers.

Activity 6.1   *Reflection*

Think back to some of your experiences in clinical practice and consider the types of leaders and managers you encountered while there. What were the characteristics of the people in charge you admired? Why did you admire these characteristics?

There are some possible answers and thoughts at the end of the chapter.

Considering the differences in the above comparisons and the answers you gave to the activity, you may start to form the opinion that leaders are better than managers in the ways in which they connect with people. You may feel that managers perhaps miss the bigger picture and are more remote and removed from the realities of practice. You may also note that some situations require management and therefore some of the key skills of management are appropriate to certain situations.

In exploring different management and leadership theories in the rest of the chapter, we hope that you will start to see, as we have already suggested, that leadership and management styles and activities can co-exist in and be practised by the same person. We further hope that you will also come to the conclusion that perhaps the art of good leadership and management is knowing what style of supervision to apply in what situation. So being a good manager may also mean being a good leader.

You may find it useful to look at the answers you gave to some of the activities in Chapter 1 (especially Activities 1.2, 1.5 and 1.6) at this point and consider what place values play in helping to shape leadership and management behaviours. Consideration of the 2010 NMC standards of proficiency, notably in the domain of 'Leadership, management and team working' competency 4 (see the start of this chapter), should be at the forefront of your mind as you read the rest of the chapter and engage with the activities and case studies it contains.

While we argue leadership and management cannot be divorced from each other, it is worth considering theories of management and theories of leadership to see what we, as nurses, can gain from them and when it might be appropriate to adopt one approach or the other in supervising care.

Theories of management

There are almost as many theories of what it is to be a manager as there are people in management positions. The purpose of the theories in this sense is to act as a guide to the key tasks and role functions of the manager. Interestingly for nursing, a profession that is increasingly driven by an emphasis on evidence-based practice, little of the work of the manager, especially the health and social care manager, is informed by any meaningful research. What this means is that we have theory and observation for guidance, but there is a large amount of scope within these theories for personal interpretation and adjustment to the individual management tasks and contexts within which these are applied. It is worth noting that there is a large amount of research into leadership and management styles and behaviours from disciplines other than nursing which can be used to inform your thinking about leadership and management and it may be worth looking at books and journals from other disciplines to inform your thinking about leadership and management practice.

In part, the lack of meaningful research into the management function is itself a product of the diversity of people, staff, managers and settings in which nurse management takes place. The uniqueness of each individual, manager, team, group and organisation, as well as the ever changing political, social and technological climate in which they work, mean it is difficult to produce research-informed strategies for management that have any real long-lasting meaning. This means that being a manager requires a constant engagement with the people being managed, the organisation and the wider political and social context.

What this implies for theories of management is that they are just that, theories. Theories are ideas about a topic which are supported by some evidence, they are not substantively proven. Even if management theories were proven, they would not all apply in the same way in every management situation.

Mintzberg's role theory

Mintzberg (1975) produced one of the most enduring descriptions of the roles of the manager. Mintzberg suggests strongly that if managers are to be effective at what they do, they need to recognise the nature and scope of the work they are undertaking and they must apply their own natural abilities to it. Mintzberg further suggests that the management role is complex and involves an intricate balance of three key roles. The power which the manager possesses arises from a recognition of their formal authority and status within the organisation. The three key roles of the manager, as Mintzberg describes them, are the interpersonal; the informational and the decisional. Within each of these roles there are a number of sub roles which taken together constitute the larger role.

Interpersonal roles:

- Figurehead – the manager performs some more basic functions which may be part of the routine of day-to-day work.
- Leader – including recruitment, staff development and motivating staff.
- Liaison – including communication with people and organisations not directly related to the immediate team.

Informational roles:

- Monitor – in this role the manager collects information about the team and the wider environment in which the team works. Some of this information comes from official sources and some from sources such as staff room gossip.

continued overleaf...

continued...

- Disseminator – involving managers sharing some of the information they have gathered from formal and informal sources from inside and outside the team with the team. There is a need for discretion here as to what information is shared, who with and when.
- Spokesperson – essentially information sharing outside of the direct team and organisation.

Decisional roles:

- Entrepreneur – the manager seeks opportunities to improve what they do.
- Disturbance handler – the manager has to respond to external pressures and make changes that have not come from within the team.
- Resource allocator – as well as managing their own time the manager allocates tasks, equipment and jobs to the team.
- Negotiator – this may mean within the team, with service users, other professions or other agencies. Sometimes this is planned; sometimes it is response to immediate pressures.

Source: Adapted from Mintzberg (1975)

What is apparent from the description of the manager Mintzberg presents is that the role requires a fair degree of adaptability on the part of the manager. Mintzberg sees the interpersonal elements of the role as being integral to the task of managing and places leadership within the description of the functions of management.

Activity 6.2 *Reflection*

Think back to your own experience of working for and with managers and try to identify when and how managers took on the different roles identified by Mintzberg. How apparent was it when they adopted a certain role? Was it clear to members of the team what the manager was doing and why?

As this activity is based on your own reflection, there is no specimen answer at the end of the chapter.

Theories such as Mintzberg's can help to add some clarity to what it is managers actually do. In Chapter 1, the case study 'The newly qualified nurse' demonstrated that the student (Julius) had little idea about what it was that the ward sister (Deirdre) did all day. Sometimes an understanding of the roles and pressures others have to work under allows us to understand better what it is they do and therefore our place in the team.

Contingency theory

Contingency theory refers to the idea that managers have to take into account a number of factors when making management decisions; that is, decisions are situation dependent. Management decisions are therefore seen as being dependent on what is happening, where it is happening and who is involved. This is perhaps best thought of as applying as much to the way in which a decision is made as to the decision that is actually made. Such an idea fits well within Mintzberg's scheme where the manager is busy juggling a number of roles in order to fulfil the task of managing.

Activity 6.3 *Critical thinking*

Think about the sort of decisions that have to be made in an emergency such as a cardiac arrest. It would seem wrong for the initial approach to be democratic: 'who would like to do chest compressions?' is rather less appropriate than saying: 'Tracy, please start chest compressions.' In other situations such as deciding who will care for which patients during a shift, it may be reasonable to allow staff to decide among themselves.

Since this is based on your own experiences, there is no specimen answer at the end of the chapter.

Contingency theory is similar to the different ways in which you will interact with clients and their relatives according to the nature of the care they are receiving, their age, mental capacity and how well you know them as individuals. As a manager, successful action relies on your understanding of a situation which in turn relies on good communication. Griffin (1999) makes the useful point that what works as a manager in one situation cannot be generalised to all such situations. As such, managers have to be adaptable to the demands of their various roles as well as the environment they work in and the people they work with.

Systems theory

Systems theory recognises that managing people, resources and care delivery requires the manager to recognise the contribution all of these elements make to the effective running of an organisation or team. Systems theorists see the world of work as a set of interdependent subsystems which interconnect to form what is a whole (or holistic) system. Von Bertalanffy (1968), the initial and most famous system theorist, recognised that systems (teams, groups, organisations) are characterised by the interactions of their components (people and their environments) and the unpredictability of those interactions.

What this means for the management of people is that the role each plays within the functioning of a team has to be recognised, supported and directed with one eye on the bigger picture. When one part of the system fails, then the whole system is affected. It is important therefore for the leader or manager to consider the role of each member of the team in achieving the team's goals.

The Hawthorne experiments (see useful websites) provide an interesting insight into how people are motivated at work by the feelings of belonging and of being paid attention to: the so called **Hawthorne effect**. Essentially the experiments undertaken at the Hawthorne factory involved making both positive and negative changes to people's working conditions and recording the impact this had on productivity. What the experiments demonstrated is that what is done is not as important as the fact that workers are being paid attention to, which alters their behaviour. A similar effect is seen in research where people react in ways which they believe a researcher wants them to because they are under scrutiny (Ellis, 2010).

Activity 6.4   *Critical thinking*

Return to Chapter 2 on teams and team working and consider the various roles that members of the team have in achieving its goals. Now consider what might happen to the wider team, system, when one member of the team fails to fulfil their role as a team member.

There are some possible answers and thoughts at the end of the chapter.

The important message for the manager here is the need to demonstrate to all members of the team that the role they play, however minor it may seem, can have a much wider impact.

Case study: The wrong mop

George is a new ward orderly who is responsible for cleaning Juniper ward. The ward has three side rooms. In side room two is a patient with methicillin-resistant staphylococcus aureus (MRSA) who is being nursed in isolation. George mops side room two and then continues to use the same mop to clean the open ward areas. Within a few days there is an outbreak of MRSA on the ward.

This case study reminds us that even the most mundane task can have a significant impact not only on the nursing team, but also the patients that we care for. The nurses on the ward may have been meticulous in their hygiene and infection control procedures when caring for the MRSA positive patient, but one component of the system, in this case George, was not and so the system, which includes the ward and the hospital at large, is affected by this single action. Of course there are a number of potential explanations for George's lack of understanding about the impact of his actions which include poor training, poor leadership or perhaps his feeling of not belonging in the ward team.

Workload management

Within the role of the manager there are a number of tasks which need to be undertaken. Some of these tasks reflect on the roles identified in the model by Mintzberg discussed earlier, others are more singular and are worthy of some discussion here.

The role of the manager in co-ordinating the work of a team was alluded to in Chapter 1, especially in the case study 'The newly qualified nurse'. The management of workload is perhaps one of the key skills for the new or aspiring nurse manager who needs to satisfy their own developmental and work-life balance needs; the needs of the team members; the needs of the organisation; and the needs of the people who use the service.

To achieve this balance the nurse manager must learn and consolidate a number of skills and, while this is not an exhaustive list, some of these skills are discussed here:

- Learn to say 'No'! The need to prioritise workloads as a manager is very real. Taking on more than you or the team can manage will mean that no one is satisfied.

- Learn to delegate. People are the greatest resource for the nurse leader and manager. Knowing your team, what they are capable of and what individuals enjoy doing means that you can delegate tasks and everyone benefits (Ellis and Abbott, 2010).

- Learn to kick the door shut. When you have a pressing task to attend to, an open door policy (which allows anyone in at any time for any reason) means you cannot concentrate on what is in front of you and so are unable to finish anything. Clearly this is not always appropriate; emergency situations may require immediate attention and shutting yourself away during a crisis is not appropriate.

- Learn to go home. If your job cannot be done in the time allotted to it, you have too much work. A tired nurse manager is likely to make mistakes and be unhappy. This is no good to anyone. Failure to achieve everything in the allotted time may also indicate the need to become more organised, delegate more effectively and manage time more wisely.

By managing their time through prioritising, saying no and sensible delegation, managers can achieve their goals and develop the team members at the same time.

Of the roles of the nurse manager, drawing up the off-duty roster is one which can often lead to disagreement and create disharmony in the team (as we saw in the case study 'The rota' in Chapter 4). For the manager who is concerned with doing things right, there are a few simple rules to follow in undertaking this task and which contribute to successful workload management. The lessons from these translate well into other management tasks.

There is a need to be open and honest about the process; people have no need to speculate, and gossip, about what they can see. An open process will involve observing two important principles: being fair and being consistent. The morally active manager is described by Dawson and Butler (2004, page 237) as acting 'on the basis of internal values, or standards, rather than (or as well as)…on the basis of externally imposed codes of conduct'. Clearly as well as being transparent in the process of work allocation it is important for the manager to allocate staff so that there are appropriate levels (the skill mix) and numbers of staff on duty at any one time.

The sorts of principles associated with moral management are also the sorts of principles associated with moral and ethical nursing practice. Fairness dictates that all staff are given equal opportunity to request days off and consistency that these are all considered according to the same criteria. Whatever tasks the manager faces, be this acting as a spokesperson or as a role model, there is a need to demonstrate moral and ethical awareness. Managers who are unable to demonstrate moral activity in their day-to-day management practice cannot reasonably require the same from their team. Moral and professional conduct is one of the cornerstones of good nursing and good management practice.

Resilience and management

One of the features of modern nursing management is the need to be resilient. Resilience is the ability to cope with, and even thrive as a result of, the stresses and challenges that being a twenty-first century nurse manager throw up. In Chapter 9, we will discuss strategies for developing confidence as a leader or manager and how this will enable you to make the transitions from student to qualified nurse and nurse leader and thereby develop the ability to cope with the challenges that nurse management and leadership create.

There are some key strategies that enable nurse managers to become more resilient and in so doing role model to their team how to cope with the challenges that nursing creates. Where a manager is able to deal with situations clearly, fairly and ethically, there will be trust within the team.

The most important strategy in being resilient is your own ability to make sense of what is happening in the world around you. In part, this ability comes from a strong understanding and belief in your core values (as discussed in Chapter 1). A positive attitude to reflecting on and learning from situations, changes and challenges is a core element of being a good nurse and later a good nurse manager.

Being positive and using new situations as opportunities to learn means in turn that you will develop problem solving abilities. The ability to solve problems means that you are in control, not only of the situation, but also of yourself. Understanding the effects of stress on yourself and on others is a key element of emotional intelligence, discussed more later, which is a necessary skill for successful managers and leaders.

Activity 6.5   *Reflection*

Consider how reflection on critical incidents throughout your training as a nurse has enabled you to make sense of some aspects of nursing practice. What strategies did you find helpful during this process? Perhaps discussion with peers, tutors, mentors or managers, reading articles, textbooks or attending lectures. How did this process help you to develop? What was it about reflection that enabled you to cope in untoward circumstances? How might these strategies translate to the need for resilience as a leader or manager?

There are some possible answers and thoughts at the end of the chapter.

Your reflections on this activity will have led you to the conclusion that being prepared emotionally and intellectually is one of the key strategies for surviving as a student, as a nurse and in the long term as a manager. As with all aspects of leadership and management, understanding your own responses to a situation will mean you are better prepared for, and more understanding of, the emotional responses of others. That is one of the fundamental requirements of effective people management.

Theories of leadership

Leadership can be regarded as one facet of the management role or as an entity in itself. It is a people focused activity that requires engagement with a team – the followers. House (2004) describes leadership as the ability to motivate and enable other people to achieve the goals of the organisation for which they work.

Being a leader can arise out of an individual's position within an organisation or team, or it may result from a natural ability a person has to inspire other people to follow them. There are a number of approaches to leadership, some of which take account of the nature of the interaction between the leader and their followers and others which take a more comprehensive view of the nature of leadership and the tasks of the leader as well as the interpersonal aspect of the role.

Transactional leadership

Transactional leadership is leadership at its most basic. As the name implies, there is a transaction taking place. The followers do what the leader asks of them in return for a reward, at its most basic a salary. The role of the leader in this model is to state what needs to be done and who will do it and then allow them to get the job done.

This approach to leadership is very much focused on getting a task done, rather than on the people undertaking the task. It is easy to imagine how this approach to leadership may be appealing when there are serious time constraints or in an emergency situation. In nursing, it does hark back to the days of task allocation when patient care was perhaps less holistic than is common today.

Relating the theory to good leadership practice, the leader who understands and communicates effectively with the team will gain the respect and trust of that team and for the team the reward for getting the job done will come from the sense of shared purpose and belonging that co-operative working brings.

Transformational leadership

Transformational leadership is about having a vision (a view of how things should or could be) and being able to communicate this idea effectively to others. The vision of how things should be may come from leaders themselves, from their managers or following discussion within a group or team. What is important about transformational leaders is that they believe, and are seen to believe, the vision.

For transformational leadership to work, there are some assumptions which need to be made and need to be true. First, people will follow a leader who can inspire them; second, a passionate leader with vision can get things done; and third, getting things done is a matter of instilling energy and enthusiasm into a group.

Transformational leadership requires there to be a relationship of trust between the leader and the follower. This trust means that the follower will do whatever it is that the leader envisions for them. As in all relationships the best way to generate trust is to show people you care about them and be consistent in your approach.

Transformational leaders succeed in what they do by having faith, not only in what they want to achieve and what they do, but also by generating and displaying trust in those they work with. Clearly one of the central focuses of the transformational leader is change. Transformational leaders who are successful in sharing their vision with their team will doubtless be able to lead their team through change more successfully than a leader who does not have the full support of the team.

It is worth thinking about whether transformational leadership is suited to health and social care, and more specifically within nursing. The simple answer to this is that the most successful nurse leaders will retain a vision of how things should be in terms of high quality and successful patient care provision. The shared values of care and compassion are the key to generating the trust which transformational leaders need in order to improve (transform) care provision.

Of course, having the faith and trust of the team is not of itself enough to make a person a transformational leader. There is also a real need for a vision that is correct and workable as well as inspiring. If we can agree that all improvement is a change, but not all change is an improvement, we can see that enthusiasm and vision without some foundation in reality is perhaps not all that helpful. Trust is generated when followers believe both that a leader cares about them as individuals and that the same leader is capable of delivering whatever it is they say they will deliver. Liking someone as an individual and trusting them as a leader are not the same thing.

Activity 6.6   *Reflection*

Think about some occasion when you have met a mentor or lecturer who you have liked because they were inspirational. Now think about whether they delivered what you expected. Did you learn what you thought you would learn? What was the difference between successful learning and less successful learning? Is a good relationship as important for learning as the content of the learning?

There are some possible answers and thoughts at the end of the chapter.

What this reflection shows is that there is more than one dimension to being an effective leader of people. Being nice is not really enough; there is a need for some substance to underpin activity.

Bass (1985), one of the leading writers on transformational leadership, suggests four essential components of effective transformational leadership. First, leaders must provide intellectual stimulation, challenging the way things are and encouraging creativity among the team. Second, they must demonstrate individualised consideration and by using good communication skills make followers feel able to share ideas and gain direct recognition for their unique contributions. Third, they need to demonstrate inspirational motivation which enables followers to experience the same passion and motivation as the leader to meet the team goals. Fourth, they need to have idealised influence; that is, they must act as a role model who followers wish to emulate while taking on the values of the leader.

Activity 6.7   *Critical thinking*

Thinking about Bass' criteria for a good transformational leader, what do you look for in a role model? How might a leader stimulate your thinking, make you feel part of something, motivate you to achieve the teams goals? Why is this important to you and how will you manage to maintain these standards throughout your nursing career?

As this is based on your own opinions and thoughts, there is no outline answer at the end of the chapter.

Adair's action-centred leadership

Adair (2010) describes leadership as being made up of three interlocking and interdependent activities (often portrayed as interconnected circles) which leaders must pay attention to in their role: the task, the team and the individual. The role of the leader is to achieve the task (in nursing this may be the provision of good quality care) through building and developing the team while developing the individuals that make up the team.

The functions of the leader as described by Adair (2010) which enable them to achieve the task are defining the task, planning how the task will be achieved, briefing the team and controlling the process. In order to achieve the task the leader also needs to pay attention to the human elements of what they are doing through evaluating, motivating, organising and providing an example to both the team as a whole and the individuals in it.

The servant leader

Many classic models of leadership identify the leader as the individual out in front with their followers coming along behind. Some modern theories of leadership take a different view of the role of leaders who have a more interdependent relationship with their team (Howatson-Jones, 2004). The role of the leader in this view is that of a leader who also has the ability to follow. This idea of the 'servant leader' is one described as an individual who wants to serve first and to whom the decision to lead comes later. Servant leaders seek leadership as a means of expanding their ability to serve.

Throughout history there have been a number of individuals who can be said to have been servant leaders. Well known examples include the Dalai Lama, Mahatma Gandhi and Mother Theresa. These individuals whose motivation lies in serving others have managed to expand their ability to do so by taking on leadership roles. While it can be argued that each of these was motivated by religion or political change, they share the common value of care for other people which is a value common to many healthcare managers and leaders.

Activity 6.8   *Critical thinking*

Think about the nurses, and other health professionals, who you have worked with and who hold positions of power. Consider those individuals you most admire. Think about what it was that you admired about them most. Consider whether they were the sort of individuals who got their hands dirty, who led by example, who seemed to lead so that they could improve the care of the people that they care for. Now think what this means for you as a nurse and how you might continue to hold the focus on patient care you have now as you progress into more senior roles.

As this is based on your own thoughts and reflections, there is no specimen answer at the end of the chapter.

What we can see from this example is that servant leadership could be a natural progression for nurses who start their career in positions where they deliver patient care. This model of leadership allows there to be some consistency in who they are and what they do as their careers progress.

This should not be seen as justification for leaders and managers who continue to deliver nursing care much of the time while neglecting the role which they are paid to perform. While we have highlighted the **person-centred** nature of health and social care this does not always mean for the leader or manager that they have to deliver face-to-face patient care. What it does mean is that they need to support their staff to do so by leading by example, providing environments conducive to learning and improving care (see Chapter 8) and by creating and supporting policies which underpin person-centred care.

The role of emotional intelligence

The concept of **emotional intelligence** has gained an increasing following over recent years. Emotional intelligence in relation to leadership and management refers to the ability of the leader or manager to understand the role that their emotions play in their decision making and the ability to recognise the emotions of the individuals within the team and how this affects the work they do (Goleman, 1996).

Recognising the influence of emotions on decision making means that leaders and managers may be in a better position to understand what motivates and what constrains staff in their work. Leaders and managers who have well developed emotional intelligence are said to be better at communicating with their team and therefore at achieving better outcomes.

Goleman (1998, page 317) defines emotional intelligence as 'the capacity for recognizing our own feelings and those of others, for motivating ourselves, and for managing emotions well in ourselves and in our relationships'. He further states that emotional intelligence is a 'learned capability'. Goleman's emotional intelligence framework comprises five elements: self-awareness, motivation, self-regulation, empathy and social skills. It is probably fair to comment that emotional intelligence is one dimension of what it is to be a good nurse and that this learned skill translates well into leadership and management roles.

It follows from this, however, that people who rely heavily on their emotions to guide their actions will tend to base their decisions on their emotional responses to a situation rather than on more objective empirical evidence and that in some situations this may be detrimental to the decisions they make (Croskerry and Norman, 2008). That said, the failure of leaders and managers to understand the role of their own emotions and those of their staff in shaping decision making and behaviours at work will mean that important issues are overlooked which may affect patient care.

Case study: The grieving staff nurse

Blossom had always been a self-confident and able staff nurse. She was friendly with staff and patients, but on the whole tended to keep herself very much to herself. Blossom had seemed a little withdrawn in recent weeks, but had said nothing to anyone until one day she went into an unexplained rage. Blossom shouted at the students and her fellow staff nurses and was rude and abrasive towards patients and visitors. Kathy, a fellow staff nurse, decided she should take control of the situation and took Blossom to one side. Blossom started to cry once in the ward office. She confided to Kathy that her father had died some weeks previously and she was finding it hard to cope.

There are two interesting elements to this case study: first, Blossom had not shared her grief with anyone and did not know how to deal with it herself; second, no one on the ward team had picked up on her distress. On two levels then emotional intelligence was seen to be lacking: in Blossom recognising the effects of grief on her behaviour and in her colleagues recognising that Blossom was grieving. Clearly, for emotional intelligence to work for leaders or managers of people, they need to develop an awareness of the effects of their own emotions before they can recognise and respond to the emotions of others.

Chapter 4 looks at emotional intelligence in the context of conflict management.

Gaining support

What we have seen in this chapter is that one of the key roles of the leader or manager in nursing is working with and through their team. In order to achieve this nurse managers and leaders need the support of their team. How this support is gained and maintained is through a mixture of good communication, good interpersonal skills and developing a sense of achievement. The team will support a leader that they trust.

Scholtes (1998) identifies trust as arising out of the feeling that leaders or managers both care for their staff and are capable of doing the job.

Figure 6.1: Trust, respect and affection

Source: Adapted from Scholtes (1998)

The model presented here demonstrates to the novice leader or manager the importance not only of getting the technical, procedural and policy elements of their role right, but also the need to take their team with them. This returns us to one of the key themes of the chapter that to be a successful nurse manager there is a clear need not only to know what you are doing, but also to nurture and develop your staff and team while you are doing it – good management and good leadership.

Chapter summary

This chapter has introduced some of the different theories of management and leadership as well as some of the ways of acting that contribute to their success. We have seen that leadership and management while often viewed as separate entities can co-exist in the same individual and that when they do they can add to the success of the manager.

This chapter has identified that some of the key values of nursing translate well into good nurse leadership and management. We have identified that for managers or leaders to be successful they need both resilience and the ability to influence people. The need for resilience clearly comes from the requirement for managers and leaders to manage what can be difficult situations, and that part of the toolkit of successful leadership and management in terms of resilience is the ability to connect with people on the human level and thereby influence what they do and how they do it.

For nurses, who enter the profession to care for others, we have suggested that maintaining the focus on care as a fundamental part of developing as a leader and manager both sets a good role model to the team and helps to develop trust. Developing trust means that nurse leaders or managers can effectively lead their team in the delivery of high quality nursing care.

Activities: Brief outline answers

Activity 6.1 (page 91)

You may remember meeting senior nurses who were able to let you know what they were doing and why you should do things in the way they wanted. Other nurses may have told you to do things because that is how things are done here. The first example is of leadership, as the senior nurse lets you see why and how you should behave in a certain way. The second example is more managerial in telling you what to do because this is policy. The best senior staff will be able to swap between being a leader and manager according to the situation and this change will appear appropriate; for example, during an emergency situation it may be best to be told what to do rather than why.

Activity 6.4 (page 95)

The failure of one part of the team to fulfil their role within the team may mean that the whole team fails to meet its goals. In terms of systems theory, this means that the system will fail not because all of the components of the system are not working, but because of the interdependence of each part of the system meaning when one part fails, the rest are all affected.

Activity 6.5 (page 97)

Using reflection as a tool and utilising the experience and understanding of others allows us to see situations in a context. Understanding the context of a situation and why things happen as they do enables us to make sense of them, and cope emotionally with things which might otherwise prove too difficult. Part of the reflection process is planning how we will meet challenges in the future, action planning, that is we become prepared. When we are prepared, we know not only how we will feel, but also how we will act and more importantly why. This means that when we meet similar situations in the future they will be less daunting. That is resilience.

Activity 6.6 (page 99)

How you feel about an individual that you have to work with or follow is often affected by whether you like them as a person and whether you feel they care about you as an individual. This is certainly an important first step in any relationship. When these same people deliver what they promise, when you learn from them what they said you would learn, it generates a feeling of great trust and gratitude. When an individual that you like is unable to deliver what they promise, you may not stop liking them, but you question whether your trust in them is well placed and you will think twice before following whatever they say in the future.

Further reading

Adair, J (2010) *Develop your Leadership Skills*. London: Kogan Page.
A really short and useful introduction to leadership as Adair sees it.

Grint, K (2002) Management or leadership? *Journal of Health Services Research and Policy*, 7 (4): 248–51.
A useful discussion of leadership and management.

Henderson, J and Atkinson, D (eds) (2004) *Managing Care in Context*. London: Routledge.
A good overview of management in health and social care.

Useful websites

www.kingsfund.org.uk/Leadership
The King's Fund – a good leadership and management resource website.

www.cipd.co.uk/subjects/lrnanddev/selfdev/emotintel.htm?IsSrchRes=1
The Chartered Institute of Personnel and Development's synopsis of emotional intelligence.

www.nhsleadershipqualities.nhs.uk/development-guide
The NHS Leadership Qualities Framework – a good overview of elements of leadership.

www.bbc.co.uk/programmes/b00lv0wx
A podcast and explanation of the Hawthorne effect which is worth listening to.

Chapter 7
Improving care, change management and entrepreneurial skills

Chapter aims

After reading this chapter you will be able to:

- compare different organisational structures;
- understand the organisations' requirements to maintain standards;
- understand change theory and its use in the change management process;
- evaluate the appraisal tools available to improve work performance;
- appreciate a new approach to changing practice through entrepreneurial skills.

Introduction

This chapter will help you understand how the organisation for which you work is structured and operates to maintain and improve standards. It looks at organisational clinical governance requirements and explores how you can work with others to plan and implement change. Included in this chapter are methods to improve standards of working through performance appraisal, supervision and 360 degree reviews. There is a section on planning, managing and implementing change to improve standards of care and service delivery. The final section looks at how entrepreneurial nurses can adopt a business minded approach to improving patient care.

Understanding your organisation

Once you have qualified, you will be busy adapting to your new responsibilities and getting to grips with a new working environment. You will have little time to think about the 'powers that be' or the 'upper echelons' of the organisational structure in which you work. But this structure has an impact on your daily working life, so it is worth spending a few minutes figuring out who controls what.

Organisations have a structure that influences the manner in which they operate and perform. The structure, which will vary according to the objectives and culture of the organisation, provides a framework for distributing responsibilities for the different departments and functions. Factors that influence the shape of this structure include size, main purpose and skills of the workforce. The historical origins of a hospital (e.g. as a Victorian workhouse) or location (in an industrial area, close to a medieval leper colony or monastery), although distant from the modern demands of current NHS or private sector healthcare, may nevertheless influence the organisation's culture.

Activity 7.1   *Evidence-based practice and research*

a. Ask your mentor if they know the origins of the organisation where you are currently on placement. Consider whether this has had any impact on the functions of the organisation today.

b. Go to the web page of the organisation and look for the welcome page. See if there is a strapline which outlines the main priorities of the organisation. There may be a statement which says 'Our main objective is to…' or 'Our mission is to…'. Finding these key messages helps you understand what the priorities are for the organisation. If there is no web page, each organisation will produce an annual report. Seek this out to see what the main priorities for the organisation are.

As this answer is based on your own research and reflections, there is no specimen answer at the end of the chapter.

An important factor in any organisational structure, whether historically derived, a private healthcare company or small scale organisation (such as a charitable foundation supporting a hospice), is the **span of control**. Used to describe the number of employees each organisation manager or head of department is responsible for, this can also be expressed in financial terms such as the budget or annual financial turnover of a department. The span of control will determine issues such as the structure, number of departments and managers in an organisation. There will usually be a leading manager, chief executive or similar post, a governing board with a number of board members, some of whom will be external to the organisation to provide expert advice or represent organisations. In the NHS, for example, these would be patient organisation and local authority representatives from the council or regional government offices.

Activity 7.2   *Evidence-based practice and research*

Find out the structure in the organisation you have a placement in or hope to work in when you qualify. Try to get hold of a copy of the structure or ask your mentor to sketch one out.

Identify who sits on the Board of the organisation as this is the main decision-making body with the power to agree or prevent service developments.

Find out if there is a nurse member of the Board who represents your professional interests.

As this answer is based on your own research and reflections, there is no specimen answer at the end of the chapter.

Organisation structure

The Learn Management website (www.learnmanagement2.com) describes five main organisational structures: tall, flat, hierarchical, centralised/decentralised and matrix. On this website you will find descriptions of each type of structure, along with their advantages and disadvantages. In brief, a tall structure is one that has many levels of management, with each line manager having a small number of people reporting directly to him or her, so that the people on the lower levels may have no contact at all with those higher up. This can have implications for accountability and communication, but it does provide employees with a clear management structure with ample opportunities for promotion.

By contrast, a flat structure has fewer management layers, but each manager has quite a large number of people (all at more or less the same level) reporting to them. This can encourage team spirit and a sense of collective belonging, but it can be difficult to manage if the organisation is large. A hierarchical organisation has much in common with a tall organisation, but there are likely to be more people reporting directly to managers on each different level, particularly at the lower levels (thus giving them a pyramid shape). The most important decisions tend to be taken by the most senior people.

The matrix structure could not be more different. In an organisation with this type of structure, the important unit is the team. Each team will be led by a project manager or team leader, and will be responsible for a specific project or aspect of the organisation's work. In some organisations, the team will only exist for the duration of the work required by the project (e.g. a team of engineers working to develop a new type of vacuum cleaner). In others, the team becomes an established department within a whole organisation structure (e.g. with responsibility for distribution of the items being made). In many cases, the matrix organisation would consist of a mixture of permanent teams and project-specific teams.

Tall structures can be contrasted with flat structures, and hierarchical organisations with matrix-based organisations. Another important contrast is between centralised and decentralised structures. In a centralised organisation, a small group of senior managers (or a 'head office', which will be in a specific location) retains the major responsibilities and powers. In a decentralised organisation, these powers are devolved down to various lower level managers, perhaps spread over a wide geographical area. Many supermarkets and chain stores are excellent examples of the decentralised structure. Each outlet is a management unit in itself, but although the manager is relatively autonomous on a day-to-day basis, he or she will be ultimately answerable to the head office – either directly or through an interim (or regional) manager.

Some organisations may find a combination of centralisation and decentralisation to be most effective. For example, functions such as accounting or warehousing may be centralised to save costs. The Department of Health uses a mixture of centralisation and decentralisation with central policy decisions being made to influence local health services. At the same time, local NHS Trusts have functions and responsibilities to respond to local population health needs and to manage their organisations according to the workforce they require to deliver those services.

Activity 7.3   *Team working*

With two or three colleagues, go to the Learn Management website and look up the various types of organisation described. Two of you can research each type and give a five minute presentation about it to the others, and then you can change roles for the next organisation type. The presentation should include one person highlighting the advantages, and the other the disadvantages. The listeners then decide whether the advantages outweigh the disadvantages, or vice versa.

When you have looked at all five organisation types, discuss as a group which model best describes the organisation in which you work.

As this answer is based on your own research and reflections, there is no specimen answer at the end of the chapter.

Nurses at board level

An influential government report in the early 1980s observed that 'If Florence Nightingale were carrying her lamp through the corridors of the NHS today she would almost certainly be searching for the people in charge' (Griffiths, 1983). In the wake of this, the RCN launched a campaign with the slogan 'Nursing should be managed by nurses' and indeed the first nurse General Managers were appointed shortly afterwards (Nursing Standard, 1985). Nurse managers should be well placed to improve the business of caring by helping boards not only to understand the quality of care patients receive on the wards, but also to make positive decisions which improve that care.

During the last two decades, the management of NHS organisations has tended to focus on financial measures and performance targets rather than on the quality of clinical care. However, the Darzi Report (Darzi, 2008) has reversed this trend, describing the improvement in quality of care as 'the basis of everything we do in the NHS'. The business of caring was brought to the forefront in the review and considered just as important as financial management.

The role of nurses at Board level in the NHS has changed and more are being appointed. The post of nurse executive (or nursing director) was established alongside the first wave of NHS trusts in 1991. In 2007 the Burdett Trust commissioned The King's Fund to develop an intensive programme of work to support executive nurses and NHS boards in raising the quality of clinical care and giving a central place to patients and how they experience healthcare.

This work has resulted in two reports:

- *From Ward to Board* (2009) sets out the key questions and findings from the first phase of the programme and identifies good practice that can be easily replicated. Key areas to be built on are identified, along with the key skills and qualities nurse executives need to fulfil their role effectively.
- *Putting Quality First: Building on 'From ward to board'* (2010) is based on observations of how nurse executives and their boards work together. This report builds on themes that emerged from the previous one, and addresses long-standing concerns about the way in which financial and administrative performance indicators have taken precedence over issues relating to the quality of clinical care.

Governance

This section examines the regulatory bodies responsible for ensuring quality and good **governance** in health and social care organisations. The White Paper *Equity and Excellence: Liberating the NHS* (DH, 2010) proposed changes to the governance, regulation and accountability arrangements of the NHS in England. The Care Quality Commission (CQC) is a regulatory body with responsibility for monitoring the quality of health and social care provision in England. It was created in 2009 through a merger of the Healthcare Commission, the Mental Health Commission and the Care Service Inspection Service. Scotland, Northern Ireland and Wales have separate governance arrangements.

Activity 7.4	*Evidence-based practice and research*

If you are in placement in an NHS organisation in England there will have been a Care Quality Commission inspection within recent years. This activity will help you find the most recent report. Go to the website **http://caredirectory.cqc.org.uk/caredirectory/searchthecaredirectory.cfm**.

continued overleaf...

continued...

In the search box put a place name or postcode and select a service you wish to find out about. You can also find out about independent nursing homes and social care providers who are registered, and therefore licensed to provide services, with the Commission.

As this answer is based on your own research, there is no specimen answer at the end of the chapter.

Case study: Investigating quality of care (CQC, 2010)

In February 2010 the Care Quality Commission investigated Cambridgeshire and Peterborough NHS Foundation Trust and warned it to improve the standards of its mental health services or face enforcement action. In December 2010 the CQC published a report which drew attention to its findings and made recommendations for improvements. The inspectors found the Trust was contravening five regulations regarding care and welfare, staffing, safeguarding people, assessing and monitoring service provision and safety and suitability of premises. The Mental Health Act Annual Statement report (2010) presented recommendations as to how the Trust should continue to conform to the Mental Health Act and Codes of Practice when detaining patients.

Some concerns identified in the 2010 review had not been fully addressed by the Trust. These were as follows:

- *Care and welfare of people who use services:*

  - *Not all care plans were person centred or included information regarding individuals' wider care and inclusion needs.*
  - *The seclusion suite on one ward is not meeting environmental requirements or the requirements of the Mental Health Act 1983 Code of Practice.*

- *Safeguarding vulnerable people who use services from abuse:*

  - *Policies in relation to adult safeguarding and incident reporting do not clearly set out arrangements that ensure consistent reporting, investigation and dissemination of learning in relation to matters regarding cases of abuse allegations and incidents.*
  - *Incident reporting and auditing systems are not robust.*

- *Safety and suitability of premises:*

  - *Poorly designed fixed furniture and the presence of potential ligature points in some parts of the premises pose a risk to people who use services.*
  - *The standard of décor and maintenance of one ward does not promote the dignity and well-being of people using services.*

- *Staffing:*

  - *There are not always sufficient numbers of staff with the right competencies knowledge, qualifications, skills and experience available to meet the needs of patients.*

- *Assessing and monitoring the quality of service provision:*

  - *Lack of consistency in grading of incidents and no safety mechanism to ensure that inconsistencies are identified and resolved.*

continued opposite...

continued...

- *Delays in the time it takes between staff reporting incidents and their managers signing off the processes (CQC, 2011).*

Although this Trust has now submitted positive action plans addressing how they plan to meet the essential standards, the CQC will be monitoring the Trust closely and will use enforcement powers if changes are not quickly brought about (CQC, 2011). This real-life case illustrates the power of the CQC and its ability to act swiftly and responsively if concerns are raised about a regulated service.

Changes to regulation

Foundation Trusts are currently regulated by Monitor, an independent regulator. Between April 2012 and April 2013, Monitor's responsibilities will be widened so that it becomes an economic regulator with responsibility for all providers of NHS care. All NHS providers will have a joint licence overseen by CQC and Monitor, with the CQC responsible for essential levels of safety and quality and Monitor responsible for ensuring continuity of essential services and financial regulation. Meanwhile, the National Institute for Health and Clinical Excellence (NICE) is developing 150 quality standards which the NHS commissioning board will develop into a comprehensive set of indicators against which quality and progress can be objectively measured.

There are also plans to implement ways of enabling the public to see how their local services are performing and have their say about the quality of care available. Local HealthWatch organisations, which will act as a voice for patients, will be funded by and accountable to local authorities and will ensure that the views of patients are reflected in the commissioning of health and social care.

Improving standards

In Chapter 5 we discussed how staff development could enable individuals to develop their skills further. Performance appraisal is one method that managers use to regulate how well individuals carry out their responsibilities. The Chartered Institute of Personnel and Development (CIPD, 2011) claims it is important to distinguish between performance management and performance appraisal. Performance management is undertaken through supervision and achievements observed against a specific set of objectives or goals, whereas performance appraisal is a dialogue between manager and subordinate to discuss an individual's performance, past and future development and the support required from the organisation and manager to achieve optimum performance. Marquis and Huston (2009) suggest the process of performance appraisal can also be a motivator towards improving performance. In this sense, performance appraisal is a tool to be used in performance management.

The CIPD (2011) recommends five key elements in the process:

1. Measurement – assessing the performance against agreed targets and objectives.
2. Feedback – providing information to the individual on their performance and progress.
3. Positive re-enforcement – emphasising what has been done well and making only constructive criticism about what might be improved.

4. Exchange of views – a frank exchange of views about what has happened, how appraisees can improve performance, the support they need from their managers to achieve this and their aspiration for their future career.
5. Agreement – jointly coming to an understanding by all parties about what needs to be done to improve performance generally and overcome any issues raised in the course of the discussion.

Appraisal tools

There are several tools that can be used for performance appraisal. The simplest is a trait rating scale where an individual is rated using a numerical score against a set of standards including their job description, knowledge, behaviours and personal traits – such as attitude to work. This method invites a subjective decision, which is open to potential bias, and, if a point scale is used, a tendency to score to the midline making the process meaningless.

Self-assessment methods involve individuals submitting a portfolio of achievements and productivity. While introspection and self-awareness can result in growth and achievement, feedback on achievements is essential for a positive result.

Management by objectives (MBO) is a technique seldom used in healthcare. It incorporates a process that negotiates both the organisation's objectives and the individual's assessments. It is a very specific form of appraisal with individuals measured against the objectives on a regular basis. In public healthcare organisations the appraisal is usually an annual event, whereas MBO is often quarterly and therefore far more intensive and orientated towards action by observable results.

Peer review is, as the name suggests, a process whereby professional colleagues monitor and assess each other's performance. It is used widely in medicine and education, and less widely in wider healthcare. The NMC uses this approach to review nursing and midwifery education. Peer review events take place on an annual basis with a group of colleagues from other, similar, organisations or professional groups conducting a review of systems and processes set against publicly available criteria. The process requires data to be collected from a variety of sources such as charts, patient care plans, information systems, other professionals, patients, etc.

An adaptation of the peer review process is 360 degree feedback. This is an assessment of performance that provides information from a variety of sources and often includes a group of colleagues that work with an individual. Usually, eight to ten people complete questionnaires that can also include a self-assessment, and which are submitted anonymously to an independent observer to collate the responses into a report for the individual. The report should demonstrate a synthesis of information about performance in a role. In healthcare, this could include patients as well as co-workers to provide all-round information which is where the name originates.

We have previously discussed clinical supervision and coaching (Chapter 5) as a means to supporting individuals develop new skills. These are also tools that a manager can utilise to improve work performance and standards.

> ## Activity 7.5   *Reflection and critical thinking*
>
> 1. How do you feel about being appraised? What are your fears and anxieties about appraisal? Think about the expectations you have. Put yourself into the shoes of the manager as well and try to understand their expectations of the process.
> 2. Consider each of the appraisal tools discussed above and draw up a table that compares the advantages and disadvantages of each method. You may need to look again at Chapter 5 on clinical supervision and coaching.
>
> *Further guidance is given on this activity at the end of the chapter.*

Rewards

Performance appraisal can also be used as a means of assessing an individual's ability to be promoted or moved to another pay band. The Knowledge and Skills Framework (KSF), defined in the Agenda for Change (AfC) pay agreement (2004), paved the way for a Gateway Policy to be formulated by NHS Trusts to ensure that staff covered by the AfC would obtain a transparent opportunity to move to a higher pay band. Under the AfC, progression from one pay point to another is assessed each year against the skills identified in the KSF bands. At defined points, known as Gateways, management decisions will be made about progression to higher levels of pay and responsibility. There are two Gateways in each of the nine pay bands: Foundation – which takes place no later than 12 months after an individual is appointed to a pay band, and Second Gateway – which is set at a fixed point towards the top of a pay band.

Planning change

You cannot have failed to notice the amount of change that has permeated the health services in recent years. These changes are sometimes driven by policies to restructure organisations, by improvements in medical science such as the development of stem cell research, or advances in society's attitudes to rights such as with the Human Rights Act (1998). In the day-to-day running of a ward or unit the types of change that take place can be personal (such as when staff change) or organisational (such as changes in shift patterns) or the way in which internal services are delivered (e.g. bed management, portering services, catering services or discharge planning methods).

There are many forces driving change in healthcare that are not just related to the UK. Rising costs of medical treatments, shortages of skilled workforces, increasing technology, availability of information and a growing elderly population have led, in some cases, to extreme destabilisation and a constant need to upgrade structures, promote better quality and manage workforce constraints. Whatever the changes to the work environment, there are those who embrace the changes and those who find it very difficult to adapt. Nurses in the future will need to be even more adaptable than they have in the past to keep up with change.

    Reflection

What is your personal perspective on change? Below is a short rating scale for you to self assess your attitude to change. Place a mark in the score that most fits your perspective: 1 = low agreement; 5 = high agreement.

	1	2	3	4	5
1. I always embrace change					
2. I look for opportunities to change things					
3. I accept change reluctantly					
4. I avoid change at all costs					
5. My response to change is the same as that of my friends and family					
6. Have you always responded to change in this way or have you changed in your lifetime?					
7. What events have altered your views and responses to change?					

As this answer is based on your own experience and reflections, there is no specimen answer at the end of the chapter.

Initiating and co-ordinating change requires well developed leadership and management skills. It requires vision and expert planning skills because vision alone is not sufficient.

Many of the best ideas for changing practice fail because of inadequate preparation and planning. Poor preparation results in problems during implementation, frustrated staff and lack of successful outcome.

Change theory

Most of the contemporary research into change management originates from the work of social psychologist Kurt Lewin in the mid-twentieth century. There are other theories; however, we will concentrate on Lewin's theory in this book and will compare it briefly with newer developments in Complexity theory and Chaos theory. If you are interested in other theories please go to the web resources for further information.

Lewin (1951) identified three stages through which change must proceed before any planned change will become embedded in an organisation or system of working. The stages are unfreezing, movement and refreezing.

Unfreezing is when the change agent proposes a convincing plan for change to the team or management. It is also when team members who are not keen on the change can be helped to draw out their anxieties or concerns about the change. At this stage people will become either discontented about the proposal or increasingly aware of the need to change. The skilful leader will be able to work with these conflicting views to build up trust in the change proposal's worth and the value of putting effort into the proposed change. Cummings and McLennan (2005) claim that an essential leadership role is to understand the different perspectives of individuals and **stakeholders** and 'to align the changes to be meaningful for them' (page 65).

During unfreezing leaders need to take account of the balance between change and stability as too much change leads to instability which results in feelings of lack of control, insecurity and anxiety. A good leader will assess the relative merits of the forces for and against change such as extent of the proposed change, nature and depth of motivation of stakeholders, and the environment in which the change will occur; this last could be physical (e.g. buildings) or political (e.g. local or national policy). The driving forces for change will need to exceed the opposing forces for change to be successful.

In the second stage there is *movement* towards accepting the change, and a plan of action and implementation is instigated. Change takes time as people adjust to the idea, come to understand the benefits of the change, and eventually become adopters of the change. Part of the planning process for change management involves including time for recognising, addressing and overcoming resistance to the proposal arising from stakeholders' attitudes, perceptions and personal values.

The final stage, according to Lewin (1951), is *refreezing*. Change needs time before it is accepted as part of the system. This means that after the change is implemented support will still be needed to embed the change. The leader's role is to help the continued integration of the change into practice to ensure refreezing – that is, the change becoming part of normal practice; if this does not occur the previous behaviours will emerge.

One method to ensure the effects of change are perceived as beneficial is to measure the outcomes of change or make improvements to the change as a result of feedback from outcome measures. Thus a plan to evaluate the change should be incorporated in the overall change management plan.

Stage 1 – *Unfreezing*

1. Gather data and information about the planned change.
2. Accurately and objectively describe the issues that are causing the problem or reason for change. Use evidence and hard facts not supposition or 'finger in the air' tactics.
3. Decide if change is really needed and identify the reasons for change. This could be a pilot for your ideas by testing on your team or one or two close colleagues.
4. Make others aware of the need for change. This also involves highlighting discontent with the current system, i.e. what is wrong or not productive. Progress to the next stage should not happen until sufficient discontent is expressed about the current system.

Stage 2 – *Movement*

1. Develop a change management plan – this could take the form of a project plan (use a **Gantt Chart** if it will help you visualise what you want to achieve – see Further reading at the end of the chapter).

continued overleaf...

continued...

2. Set goals and objectives.

3. Identify areas of support and resistance.

4. Include everyone who will be affected by the change in its planning; however, you may want to have a small project group or reference group to help manage the project with you.

5. Set target dates and timelines.

6. Develop appropriate strategies.

7. Implement the change.

8. Be available to support others and offer encouragement through the change process.

9. Use strategies for overcoming resistance to change.

10. Evaluate the change.

11. Modify the change if necessary.

Stage 3 – *Refreezing*

Support others so that the change is sustainable and remains in place to achieve improved outcomes.

Figure 7.1: Steps of Change
Source: Adapted from Marquis and Huston (2009) page 171.

Case study: Change management

Cummings and McLennan (2005) outlined four steps in a change management project to introduce advanced practice nurse roles into a traditionally, medically orientated tertiary care oncology centre. Their main aim was to engage stakeholders in the change process and use an evidence-based approach. Step one was to identify a change model to guide the project. They did this by using Lewin's theoretical change model and adapting it to connect action research and policy drivers for change. The policy drivers challenged stakeholders' values and beliefs (i.e. the value of advanced nursing) and competence, standards of practice, financial savings, medical and nursing workloads.

The second step was to assign a 'champion' or change agent to the project to work closely with staff through the unfreezing stages of the project and enable the final stage which is beyond the change itself. In the third step a forum was created, involving members from all the professional groups involved in the change, to facilitate open communication between everyone who would be affected by the change and change process. The final stage was to support staff through and beyond the change process to ensure the change became embedded into the working practices of the team.

Cummings and McLennan (2005) found that multidisciplinary team work, already established in the unit, was an important lever to help implement and embed the change. You will have noticed that all the way through the change process communication of intentions and plans, which ensures individuals and teams are engaged and informed in the change plan, has been paramount to creating an effective change strategy.

Activity 7.7   *Decision making*

Identify a change you would like to make in your personal life. List the driving forces that you think are your reasons for wanting to change. Then list the restraining forces that you think will inhibit you making the change. Work out a plan, utilising all of the steps of change in Figure 1 above, to achieve the change.

Hint

Remember the driving forces will need to exceed the restraining forces (Beckhard and Harris, 1987) and you will need to feel sufficient discontent with how things currently are for the change process to tip from unsuccessful to successful. You will also need to plan time for the change to be embedded into your everyday life. This means it will take longer than you originally planned; especially if you were hoping for quick results.

As this answer is based on your own decision-making, there is no specimen answer at the end of the chapter.

Complexity theory and chaos theory

Lewin's change theory is a linear approach to change with an optimistic view that change once implemented will be refrozen and equilibrium re-established. In this current world, where science is moving the frontiers of knowledge forward at an increasing pace and organisations respond to change more rapidly, the linear approach has been found wanting. This is particularly evident in UK healthcare where long-term planning is problematic due to fluctuating economic and political influences. Consequently, non-linear change theories such as complexity theory and chaos theory now influence contemporary change theory.

Complexity theory maintains that we inhabit a complex world where individuals are multifaceted and situations are forever dynamic and changing. The theory originates from physics where the natural order of science is challenged by systems that are constantly adapting because of the interaction between parts and feedback loops that change things and do not maintain the status quo. An example of this is that an individual may have behaved in a certain way in the past but their future behaviour may not be predictably the same.

Olson and Eoyang (2001) developed a theory of complex adaptive systems which maintains that we should not focus on the large changes taking place but on the effects of change at a micro level between individuals. It is at the individual level where relationships, and simple expressions of rules, are responsible for change. When applying this theory to changes in healthcare it suggests we should concentrate on the individuals who work in the organisations and understand these relationships before attempting to unfreeze as in Lewin's theory. They also suggest that continual monitoring and adaptation is needed for refreezing to be achieved.

Research summary: Complexity theory and organisations

Anderson, Corazzini and McDaniel (2004) undertook a study, underpinned by complexity theory, to analyse the effects of organisational climate and communication patterns on high staff turnover in nursing homes. They surveyed 3,449 employees in 164 randomly

continued overleaf...

continued...

selected nursing homes in North Carolina, USA, to identify the perceptions of staff about organisational climate and communication. They also asked questions about the characteristics of the homes' facilities, allocation of resources and turnover. The results were analysed statistically using a hierarchical regression technique (to examine the relationship between variables).

They found that there was a lower turnover in the lower paid staffing groups (which had the highest overall turnover rates) when the climate was viewed positively and communication was open. Where there was a reward-based climate and high levels of open communication, staff performed better than in those homes with unclear and confusing communication methods. They also found where there were good levels of staffing, and senior staff who had been in position for a long time, there was more likely to be lower staff turnover. Thus, a stable leadership situation enhanced staff satisfaction with workplace conditions through the influence of the leadership style. A reward themed climate and open communication were aspects of this style.

Chaos theory was first described in 1960 by Edward Lorenz, a meteorologist working on the problem of weather predictability. It is related to complexity theory in that it refers to the unpredictable and adaptive factors that affect events. Lorenz discovered that a minor change in a part of an experiment could change the whole outcome. A practical example is where a slight rise in the temperature of the ocean in one place in the world may have an effect on the airflow that will eventually lead to a change in temperature in another part of the world.

Chaos theory is a new science that helps us understand why a small change in a situation can alter how a system functions. Chaos theory also suggests that it is impossible to know what this change may be because there are so many different variables that can affect a situation. For example, if you know everything about football, the players, strategies, ground conditions and everything involved, you still cannot accurately predict the outcome. Yet, if you watch repeated games you would be able to predict some elements of the game.

The application of complexity theory to change management in organisations provides a means to understand why change does not always go to plan because of unpredictable multifactorial influences and, secondly, that understanding small effects, as chaos theory suggests, can have a big effect in a change management plan. For example, individuals who do not trust the change plan or do not think it can work could jeopardise the change plan. However, if they are brought into the change process and their ideas given a hearing they may not feel the need to jeopardise the plan. A major lesson for managers is that they cannot completely control a change plan because there will always be some elements that cannot be predicted in advance that will affect it. Managers need to learn how to manage the anxiety that accompanies change as well as flexibility and the ability to think on their feet so that they can manage the unexpected.

Living in a constantly changing world where there is rapid technological, social, cultural and political change, we have to be prepared to adapt, be willing to learn and test our assumptions. Things that worked in the past may not work in the future and nurses have always been able to find new ways of managing problems and being creative. That is why in the next section we will explore how nurses can use this creativity to improve patient care.

Tools for change: Entrepreneurship

In 2004 the International Council of Nurses (ICN) produced a monograph that gives guidance on the scope for nurses to become self-employed using expert skills and knowledge. In the UK there has been limited uptake of independent practitioners of nursing and midwifery; however, the skills of entrepreneurship are now being debated as a potential, valuable contribution to innovative healthcare initiatives. The ICN sets out how this can be understood by describing three different types of nursing entrepreneur:

- Entrepreneur: An individual who assumes the total responsibility and risk for discovering or creating unique opportunities to use personal talents, skills and energy and who employs a strategic planning process to transfer that opportunity into a marketable service or product.
- Nurse entrepreneur: A proprietor of a business that offers nursing services of a direct care, educational, research, administrative or consultative nature. The self-employed nurse is directly accountable to the client, to whom, or on behalf of whom, nursing services are provided.
- Nurse intrapreneur: A salaried nurse who develops, promotes and delivers an innovative health/nursing programme or project within a given healthcare setting based upon the skills of entrepreneurism (ICN, 2004).

It is this latter role that we will be exploring in this chapter. Within these definitions it is clear that the only difference between an intrapreneur and entrepreneur is the setting in which the skills of entrepreneurship are used.

To understand the influence of entrepreneurism on the concept of intrapreneurism we need to consider its antecedents. There is no commonly accepted definition of the terms 'entrepreneur' and 'entrepreneurship' and furthermore the meaning is shifting as it is applied to healthcare endeavours as intrapreneurism. In business or commercial terms it is someone who has a new idea and wishes to undertake a new venture with a responsibility for the risks that may result and the outcome. There is an implicit sense that the entrepreneur will personally gain from the venture. An entrepreneur will see opportunities for developments and take advantage of those opportunities; they can act as a catalyst for change and research, innovation, introducing new technologies, increasing efficiency, productivity, and generate new products or services. An intrapreneur will essentially do the same but within the confines of an organisation and will benefit less from the outcomes but will also be exposed to less attendant risk.

Traynor et al (2006) (see Further reading section at the end of this chapter) reported on a research project that investigated the extent and potential for entrepreneurial activity in nursing, midwifery and health visiting (NMHV). In 2007, Drennan et al published the findings and claimed that, while they found a range of NMHV entrepreneurial activity in the UK, there is very little in relation to the total numbers of nurses, midwives and health visitors registered in the UK. This reflects the international picture. The examples of nurse entrepreneur activity that were found involved nurses being creative and flexible in their working environments to solve problems or substituting for medical roles. The researchers found that nurses in certain fields (such as public health or specialist nursing) were more likely to have carried out entrepreneurial activity. Specific examples of activity were found through knowledge transfer (through training and consultancy), invention of healthcare products and small business provision of infrastructure services to healthcare and self-employed and small business provision of direct healthcare services.

The study attempted to find a relationship between entrepreneurial activity and patient choice but found this to be weak except in the case of independent midwifery. Yet in 20 per cent of the documents they analysed this was an aspiration along with seeking autonomous practice and achieving personal and professional accomplishment. Financial incentives were not a prominent feature; however, this was not borne out by seminar participants who felt that financial gain was a hidden agenda due to the lack of a commercial culture within the NHS.

Activity 7.8 — *Skills development*

Think of an area of practice, service delivery or patient care that you would like to see improved. Imagine you are going to present this idea to a *Dragons' Den* (BBC TV programme) type panel of peers. (If you are not familiar with *Dragons' Den* please generate an idea for presentation to a panel of peers.)

1. Who would you have on the panel? What skills and knowledge would you expect them to have to make a decision about your idea?
2. Design a simple presentation that 'sells' your idea to the panel.

Hint

Go to the BBC web page **http://news.bbc.co.uk/1/hi/business/2943252.stm** which will give you tips on writing a business plan.

As this answer is based on your own research and reflections, there is no specimen answer at the end of the chapter.

The debate is still open on whether or not entrepreneurialism can drive forward a culture of innovation and creativity benefiting patient care. There remain several obstacles, such as the prevailing ideology of the NHS as a public sector organisation and therefore by default a 'not for profit industry' and the socialisation of NMHVs that does not include a business frame of reference. As Drennan et al (2007) point out, there has been no systematic measurement of the outcomes of NMHV enterprise activities to support the effectiveness of entrepreneurial activity. Yet there are examples of where it has made a difference (Drennan et al, 2007).

Chapter summary

In this chapter we have examined different organisational structures that you can map out in your own organisations. You can then identify where the decisions are made in your organisation which will, in turn, help you understand where to find information about the decisions. Nurses are playing an increasingly pivotal role in organisational decisions as government policy recognises that nurses can represent not only their profession but also the patient's point of view. We have studied the governance requirements for NHS institutions to ensure they are meeting the standards required and also looked at the

continued opposite...

continued...

regulatory arrangements starting in 2012. While looking at standards we considered how to improve care on a personal level through performance appraisal and compared some of the methods that can be used. The chapter has also looked at the theory underpinning change management and contemporary theory developments. Change management is a huge subject and we have only briefly touched on the change planning process to raise your awareness of the methods available. Finally, we looked at the potential for a newer approach to introducing change and improving standards with an emphasis on social enterprise and entrepreneurial skills.

Activities: Brief outline answers

Activity 7.5 (page 113)

1. Preparation for appraisal is the best method of ensuring levels of anxiety are minimised on the part of both the appraisee and the appraiser. This means ensuring the method and purpose of the appraisal are clearly articulated and agreed beforehand, standards are transparent and evident in the organisation's policies, strengths as well as weaknesses are explored and the paperwork is available and prepared in advance by both parties. Further support for conducting appraisals can be found on the CIPD website listed in the Useful websites section below.

2. Comparison of appraisal methods:

	Advantages	**Disadvantages**
Clinical supervision	Personal and focused Deeper trusting relationship can be established Can specifically match specialty area to improve performance	Could become too intense Personalities may not match More resources required for time
Coaching	Personalised Identifies specific goals Enhances personal motivation	Takes time Needs in-depth coaching training to be effective
Trait rating scales	Uses a set standard that is transparent Incorporates personal behaviours such as attitudes	Can lead to subjective assessments Central tendency in scores 'Halo' or 'horns' effects from rater
Self-appraisal	Collects examples of impact on standards and is achievement orientated Enables personal growth and awareness	Gives little scope for feedback – positive or negative May have focused on goals that do not correspond to organisational targets for improvement

continued overleaf...

continued...

Management by objectives	Determines individual progress incorporating both employee and organisation's goals Promotes individual growth and excellence	Authoritarian and directive managers find this approach difficult due to the negotiated nature of the goal setting Some employees may set easily achievable goals
Peer review	Has the potential to increase accuracy of performance appraisal as collects data from wider range of sources Can enhance team working and improve understanding between different teams, especially interdisciplinary disciplinary teams Provides increased opportunities for professional learning and sharing of good practice	Requires high levels of trust to share data More time consuming than one-to-one appraisals Takes time to orientate staff to the process, requires training and has high administration costs Shifts authority away from manager which can be threatening to the manager who may feel exposed
360 degree appraisal	Feedback from a variety of sources Provides a broader perspective on an individual's performance	Requires questionnaires to be designed and administered, data collected anonymously and collated into a report which is costly and time consuming Could be threatening to have such a wide selection of subjective opinions about an individual's performance

Further reading

Dwyer, J, Stanton, P and Thiessen, V (2004) *Project Management in Health and Community*. London: Routledge.

Gantt, HL (1910) *Work, Wages and Profit*, published by *The Engineering Magazine*, New York; republished as *Work, Wages and Profits*. Easton, PA: Hive Publishing Company, 1974.

Kritonis, A (2004) Comparison of Change Theory. *International Journal of Scholarly Academic Intellectual Diversity*, 8 (1).

Marquis, BL and Huston, CJ (2009) *Leadership Roles and Management Functions in Nursing: Theory and Applications*. Philadelphia, PA: Lippincott, Williams and Wilkins, Chapter 24: Performance Appraisal.

Traynor, M, Davis, K, Drennan, V, Goodman, C, Humphrey, C, Locke, R, Mark, A, Murray, SF, Banning, M and Peacock, R (2006) *A Report to the National Co-ordinating Centre for NHS Service Delivery and Organisation Research and Development of a Scoping Exercise on 'The Contribution of Nurse, Midwife and Health Visitor Entrepreneurs to Patient Choice'.*

Yoder-Wise, PS (2007) *Leading and Managing in Nursing* (4th edition). St Louis, MO: Mosby Elsevier, Chapter 16: Leading Change.

Useful websites

www.cipd.co.uk/hr-resources/factsheets/performance-appraisal.aspx
Performance appraisal: Chartered Institute of Personnel and Development Performance Appraisal; guidance and processes.

www.learnmanagement2.com
Organisation structures: The Learn Management website gives lots of theory and useful explanatory diagrams.

www.scottlondon.com/interviews/wheatley.html
The New Science of Leadership: An Interview with Margaret Wheatley by Scott London.

www.bbc.co.uk/programmes/p00548f6
Chaos theory: BBC broadcast of radio programme chaired by Melvyn Bragg in 2002 with Susan Greenfield, Senior Research Fellow, Lincoln College, Oxford University, David Papineau, Professor of the Philosophy of Science, King's College, London, and Neil Johnson, University Lecturer in Physics at Oxford University, discussing chaos theory. The broadcast explains chaos theory and its roots and application to modern day usage. You will need Realplayer software to listen to the broadcast, which lasts for 45 minutes.

www.rcn.org.uk/__data/assets/pdf_file/0018/115632/003215.pdf
Becoming an entrepreneur: RCN guidance on becoming an entrepreneur and running your own business.

www.nurse-entrepreneur-network.com
USA Nurse Entrepreneur Network web page: Advice and tips on setting up a nursing business.

www.youtube.com/watch?v=ZxuwVqyyrmM
Wendy Miles Entrepreneurial nurse 'Nurse Joey': Example of a nurse entrepreneur success that has improved nurses' working lives, benefited the organisation and released time for patient care. Wendy developed a handy pocket-like pouch to assist nurses; it saves time for nurses to carry small essential equipment about with them while they work.

www.entreprenurses.net/
Entreprenurses: A website for UK nurses wishing to learn more about developing entrepreneurial skills and links to short learning modules, podcasts and relevant literature.

Chapter 8
Creating a learning environment

NMC Standards for Pre-registration Nursing Education

This chapter will address the following competencies:

Domain 1: Professional values

7. All nurses must be responsible and accountable for keeping their knowledge and skills up to date through continuing professional development. They must aim to improve their performance and enhance the safety and quality of care through evaluation, supervision and appraisal.

Domain 3: Nursing practice and decision-making

1. All nurses must use up-to-date knowledge and evidence to assess, plan, deliver and evaluate care, communicate findings, influence change and promote health and best practice. They must make person-centred, evidence-based judgements and decisions, in partnership with others involved in the care process, to ensure high quality care. They must be able to recognise when the complexity of clinical decisions requires specialist knowledge and expertise, and consult or refer accordingly.

Domain 4: Leadership, management and team working

1. All nurses must act as change agents and provide leadership through quality improvement and service development to enhance people's well-being and experiences of healthcare.

5. All nurses must facilitate nursing students and others to develop their competence, using a range of professional and personal development skills.

Essential Skills Clusters

This chapter will address the following ESCs:

Cluster: Care, compassion and communication

1. As partners in the care process, people can trust a newly registered graduate nurse to provide collaborative care based on the highest standards, knowledge and competence.

   At entry to the register:

   14. Uses professional support structures to develop self awareness, challenge own prejudices and enable professional relationships, so that care is delivered without compromise.

4. People can trust a newly qualified graduate nurse to engage with them and their

continued opposite...

· · *continued...* ·

family or carers within their cultural environments in an acceptable and anti-discriminatory manner free from harassment and exploitation.

At entry to the register:

13. Through reflection and evaluation demonstrates commitment to personal and professional development and life-long learning.

Cluster: Organisational aspects of care

12. People can trust the newly registered graduate nurse to respond to their feedback and a wide range of other sources to learn, develop and improve services.

At entry to the register:

8. As an individual team member and team leader, actively seeks and learns from feedback to enhance care and own and others professional development.

18. People can trust a newly registered graduate nurse to enhance the safety of service users and identify and actively manage risk and uncertainty in relation to people, the environment, self and others.

At entry to the register:

9. Reflects on and learns from safety incidents as an autonomous individual and as a team member and contributes to team learning.

10. Participates in clinical audit to improve the safety of service users.

Chapter aims

After reading this chapter you will be able to:

- explain what an environment of care is;
- identify what a learning environment is;
- explain why a learning environment is important;
- discuss how a learning environment might be created.

Introduction

Nursing, in common with all health and social care, is evolving. In great part this evolution is driven by the society and culture that we live in and by the changing technology we work with as well developing understandings of the nature and experience of care. Within this changing environment there is a need for nursing, and individual nurses, to keep pace with developments. The increased professionalisation of nursing, clearly demonstrated by the move to an all graduate profession, further requires nurses to be engaged with their own development and learning in order to meet the demands of twenty-first century care provision.

Learning and developing are therefore constant and enduring requirements for all nurses and the need to facilitate this is a key function of nurse leaders and managers. This chapter describes how the creation and maintenance of a learning environment in the clinical setting can contribute to the development of nurses and nursing. You will be challenged within this chapter to consider what this means for you as an individual, as well as how you might take the messages contained in it forward in your career as a leader or manager of nurses.

What are 'environments of care'?

Before we go on to consider what is meant by 'a learning environment', it is worth taking a moment to consider what is meant by the term environments in the sense used here. Environments refer to many things including the physical nature of a building and its surroundings as well as the meanings different people attach to the same physical space.

Activity 8.1 *Reflection*

To understand the ways in which different people attach different meanings to spaces, let's begin by reflecting on the nature of the work environment. When you are working in the hospital setting consider the different ways in which people may view the area in which you work. Consider how you see the area, how the permanent staff see it, how visiting staff see it, how patients see it and how patient visitors see it. What are their different interpretations based on? Why is this important? If you do not work in the hospital setting, consider the same questions in the context of the area in which you do work.

There are some possible answers and thoughts at the end of the chapter.

The interpretation of what an environment is, using the answers to the reflection, very much hinges on the function of the area concerned and your role in relation to that function. Different people see the same area in a different light and have different views about the nature and workings of the same place. This gives us some clues as to what an environment of care is about, but this is not the whole story.

Environments, especially care environments, are very much the product not only of what goes on there, but the ways in which people behave and interact. In this sense environments can be considered to reflect the psychosocial nature of a place. Many commentators refer to environments as 'cultures' (Handy, 1993) and in many ways this term is as useful as environments, if not more so; this is because the word culture conjures up an image of something more ingrained, natural and all encompassing than the term environment.

The psychosocial feel of a ward, clinical area or team is closely related to the ways in which the people there talk to and about each other, the way in which they interact with people who are visitors to the area, the general ambience if you like. In many respects, the environment or culture (we will use the terms interchangeably) created in a care area reflects the values of the people who work there.

As nurses, and especially as leaders or managers, we have the ability to affect the environment in which we work. Understanding the impact we have as individuals and as leaders and managers is essential to understanding how to manage environments; you may find it useful to revisit the

Johari window discussed in Chapter 1 at this stage to remind yourself about how others see us and how we see ourselves and what impact this has on relationships.

As a leader of people, the tone and nature of your interactions with others will set the benchmark by which others act. If you are seen not to care about where you work, or the people who work there, neither will the team. If you are brash, loud or condescending, then members of the team will be too. It is almost impossible to overestimate the impact that a leader has on their immediate environment. The message about the impact of the leader on the environment of the team they lead is therefore clear; in most instances leaders create the culture.

The NMC (2002) states that lifelong learning 'requires an enquiring approach to the practice of nursing and midwifery, as well as to issues which impact on that practice'. The role of the manager and leader in developing environments of care that support such learning development is critical. Creating a learning culture is something that a leader must therefore do by setting an example, not only in undertaking formal education, but by learning from their team, their clients, from complaints and from their own practice.

Lee et al (2010, page 475) state: 'By practising the knowledge builder role, leaders create opportunities and processes that stimulate and encourage knowledge sharing amongst team members.' This knowledge building role is achieved by offering new ideas and solutions to problems and by encouraging dialogue in the team. The key message here is that, for a team to develop a learning culture, the leader or manager must take the lead.

What a learning environment is

A learning environment is essentially a set of attitudes, values and their corresponding actions that creates a culture in which learning and development can take place. Quinn (1995) suggests the learning that takes place in the clinical setting is more meaningful to nursing students than that which occurs in the classroom setting. The proposal here is that the opportunities for learning and development which occur in the clinical setting are invaluable to the development of students. We would argue that this point can be stretched further to include all of the staff who work in a particular setting.

A ward, clinic or community team whose members are empowered to learn and develop will be able to provide meaningful care which not only reflects current clinical trends but which puts the patient at the heart of care. A team which operates in a learning environment will seize every opportunity to grow and develop and as a result their ability to care will be enhanced. In this sense, a learning environment is one which fosters positive development and change.

Bersin (2010, page 16) argues that a learning environment is 'the collective practices that encourage sharing of information and all forms of people development'. This idea further supports the idea that learning is more than an optional extra within the team; it is fundamental to the development of all members of the team and therefore the improvement of what they do. As such the creation, adoption and maintenance of a learning environment is a fundamental approach to addressing the standards of proficiency highlighted at the start of the chapter. What this means for you as an individual student or nurse will be discussed later in the chapter.

Why learning environments are important

Increasing emphasis is being placed on the benefits associated with work-based learning in today's health and social care provision. In some part, this is evidenced by the increase in the number and range of foundation degrees available and in the increasing provision of workplace learning modules in post-registration continuing professional development programmes for health and social care professionals.

The emphasis on work-based learning has been described by Spouse (2001) as arising from the need to generate workers who have moved on from being skilled and technically competent to becoming active problem solvers who are able to adapt and develop in tandem with their environment.

Developing a learning environment in the workplace has the potential to bring many benefits to the team and to the individuals within the team. A team established in a learning culture can rapidly adapt to change and develop new ways of working that are consistent with best practice. Staff who work in and adopt the values of a learning organisation both feel and are more empowered to do their job and as a consequence have the ability to be more effective at what they do.

Activity 8.2   *Reflection*

Reflect on the times in the classroom setting when you have engaged with the conversation around whatever it is you were learning. How did your engagement in the debate around the topic affect your learning? Did your contribution have an impact on what you learnt and how you felt about what you learnt?

There are some possible answers and thoughts at the end of the chapter.

Your answers to the above reflection probably demonstrate that on the occasions you engaged in what was happening in the classroom you learnt more, felt happier and were clearer about the subject matter. What is more important is that engaging in what is going on probably helped you to feel more involved, part of something if you like, as well as feeling you contributed to the learning and development of the group as a whole.

Certainly the same ideas translate into the practice setting where engaging in learning, rather than being the passive recipient of knowledge, will greatly affect the learning which you are able to take from a situation. Consider this scenario:

Case study: The same mentor

Paul is a student nurse in his first year of training. Paul has a clinical placement on a care of the elderly ward and is not at all happy with it as there is not enough high tech care going on. Paul comes in to work each shift, as he knows he must, and goes through the motions of caring for the elderly patients. He washes and helps to feed patients but does little in the way of communication and does not attempt to understand the care needs of those he nurses. Paul's mentor offers little in the way of teaching, support or advice to Paul. Overall, it is a pretty poor experience and Paul does little more than endure it.

continued opposite...

---

continued...

Mary, also a first year student, is placed on the same ward as Paul. Mary is keen to understand the care she is giving and what it means for the patients. She too would prefer to work somewhere more exciting but has decided to get what she can in the way of learning from her experience. Mary talks to her patients and asks them about their lives. She observes them closely when washing and dressing them and takes note of issues such as the development of pressure areas. Mary listens when patients explain their symptoms and makes mental notes to look things up when she is off duty. Mary asks questions of her mentor and explores ideas and tries to understand the new experiences she is having. Mary's mentor is the same person mentoring Paul, but offers Mary different learning opportunities and looks for ways to enhance her learning experience. Mary quite quickly starts to enjoy her placement and learns a lot about good quality nursing care provision.

This case study may reflect some of the experiences you have had either as a student or a mentor. What is important to understand in this case study is the learning opportunities for both Mary and Paul are the same. What makes the difference is their approach to learning. Mary adopts a positive and open approach to learning. You might say she embodies a learning culture in herself, and as a result she gets a lot from her experience. Paul on the other hand closes himself off to learning and therefore gets little from his placement.

The reward for Mary in adopting this positive approach to her own development is enjoyment of the placement and enhanced learning. It is clear her mentor also gained something from mentoring Mary and therefore sought opportunities to support her development.

As well as the opportunities that arise for self development, learning cultures bring other rewards to the team and the organisation at large. Consider again the case study above. In being more diligent about her care provision and in seeking not only to provide care but to understand the care she is giving, Mary has the opportunity to identify and prevent some potential complications arising in the patients she cares for. Such proactive nursing will benefit Mary, her patients and the team and wider organisation in reducing complication rates and the time patients stay in hospital.

From the perspective of the ward manager the constructive approach to learning Mary has adopted demonstrates benefits for the team in the creation of a positive environment. For the team leader or ward manager the fostering of a positive learning culture will benefit the team in helping with staff recruitment and retention as well as the potential reduction in absences from work.

What is fascinating about this is the impact that allowing people to ask and answer questions can have on both morale and clinical outcomes. It seems so insignificant a thing to do, but clearly the effect is great.

Elements of the learning environment

So far we have identified a definition of a learning culture and have explored some of the benefits for the individual, team and organisation. In order to better understand the notion of learning environments it is now worth exploring the elements which go towards creating and sustaining them.

Peter Senge (1990), one of the leading writers on learning organisations, identifies five key elements – he calls them disciplines – which need to be in place for a learning organisation to be generated and maintained.

1. **Systems Thinking** – this is essentially the ability to see the bigger picture. Seeing the big picture is an important element of nursing and leadership because of the complex nature of caring for people. Jackson and Ellis (2010) argue that whole systems thinking in complex environments requires us to: identify all of the components of the system (people) and their roles as well as the nature of the interrelationships between them; recognise that working in a whole system is beneficial and understand the risks of whole systems working. The idea is that we see the interconnectedness of what each component (individual) of the system does and work to maximise its input (in much the same way as we explored team working in Chapter 2 and in Chapter 7 when we explored systems theory).

2. **Personal Mastery** – this is about the commitment of the people in the system to self development. Self development in this sense is about realising our potential and striving to be the best that we can be through constant and consistent self development – clearly this relates to the exercise of our personal values as we explored in Chapter 1.

3. **Mental Models** – requires that we identify and acknowledge the values, issues and beliefs that prevent us from being all we can be. This process involves reflection on ourselves and our motivations and becoming open and receptive to new ideas and ways of working; this often requires a change in both personal and team cultures.

4. **Building Shared Visions** – for the leader or manager this is about gaining consensus on the view of how things should be from all of the members of the team. When the team can agree to a vision of how things should be they can work consistently and supportively to achieve it. As well as understanding your values, as a leader you will need to understand and acknowledge the values of the team.

5. **Team Learning** – this is the final and fundamental aspect of creating a learning culture. One person does not make a culture alone. Nursing involves the co-operative working of nurses and other care professionals. Learning together facilitates the creation of relationships which enable the wider team to work together more effectively.

The Five Disciplines needed to create a learning environment
Source: Adapted from Senge (1990).

What Senge's model demonstrates is that the creation of learning cultures requires the ability to see how things fit together, personal commitment, a change in thinking, shared drive and a willingness to learn together. So some of the messages here are about us as individuals and others about us and the way we interact in, or lead, teams.

Senge (1996) further identifies that the first step on the road to becoming a learning team or organisation is a willingness to allow people of all levels to lead in different ways. This requirement points to the need for each individual within the learning environment to commit to the values and practice of learning together.

What this means for you

The teams that work within a learning environment are made up of many individuals. As we have discussed, to a great extent the culture of the team derives from the actions and values of the leader or manager. The message is therefore clear for the leader or manager who wants to create a learning culture: lead by example. But what if you are not the manager or leader? What do the messages of this chapter hold for you?

As with all aspects of leading and managing, the first port of call is self. We saw in Chapter 4 that to effectively deal with conflict you must first of all ensure you are not the problem; we saw in Chapter 1 that to be an effective leader you must first know yourself and what drives and motivates you. Similarly, if you want to develop into the sort of leader who can promote learning and development, you must first of all develop yourself. Such development is not all about learning new things and ideas; it is more about your attitude to learning and development – or your values. For the student nurse this may mean adopting a more proactive approach to learning. You have made an important first step in choosing to read books such as this. If you are a trained nurse your attitude to your own continuing professional development is equally important.

Not only is your attitude to self development important, but so too is your attitude to the learning and development of others. Are you happy to share what you know? Do you support colleagues and friends who need to understand something that you already know? Are you willing to listen to and learn from others, perhaps even those you consider to be more junior to yourself? Are you comfortable in asking questions?

Activity 8.3 _Reflection_

Consider the questions in the paragraph above. How do you approach a situation where you know little about what is going on? What do you do when you encounter a new disease or a new way of managing the signs or symptoms of disease? How do you really feel about learning from patients or other staff? What are the values you have which underpin this answer?

As this is based on your own observations, there is no specimen answer at the end of the chapter.

There are some key challenges here about the way in which you present yourself to others as well as understanding what truly motivates you and your practice. Certainly the culture of the place in which you work will impact on how you answer and how you behave, but once again the onus rests with you as to how you will react to new challenges. For the leader, again the message about leading by example is clear; if you are comfortable to ask questions and develop your understanding so will your staff be; if you make people feel valued when they ask questions then they will ask questions.

Developing a learning environment – the challenge

Now we have some understanding of the nature of learning environments, their benefits to the individual, team and wider organisation, the challenge is to understand for ourselves how we might create and develop such an environment . For the remainder of this chapter, this challenge takes the form of a series of activities which set out to help you identify your orientation to learning environments, your experience of learning environments to date and your understanding of how a learning environment might be created.

It is important that you explore these issues in order to address the requirement of the 2010 NMC Standard of proficiency: Leadership, management and team working, number 5: 'All nurses must facilitate nursing students and others to develop their competence, using a range of professional and personal development skills.'

Activity 8.4   *Reflection*

Reflecting on how you feel about learning in general and learning within the practice setting in particular will say something about your orientation to learning environments. Consider these questions and answer truthfully. You may find some of the comments from mentors in your practice assessment document will help you to identify how others perceive your learning behaviours:

- How do you feel about new situations in the practice setting?
- Do you like new experiences or are you only comfortable with things that you know?
- How do you feel about asking questions?
- Does it matter who you are asking the questions of?
- Are you comfortable to ask questions in front of others?
- When asked a question that you do not know the answer to by a patient do you make up an answer, say you don't know and find someone else or tell them that you will find out?
- When you come across something that you do not understand do you ignore it, ask questions of people that do, go away and look it up for yourself, ask questions and look it up?

As this is based on your own observations, there is no specimen answer at the end of the chapter.

What these questions will help you to appreciate is what you value in the way of learning and understanding in the clinical setting. While there are no wrong answers as such, primarily because these questions do not ask you what is the right thing to do but ask you what it is YOU do, there are some states of behaviour and responses which are perhaps more in line with the values needed to engage in a learning environment.

What is needed from you in terms of engaging in self development which makes you fit for lifelong learning and engagement in, and potentially future creation of, learning environments is: keenness to engage in and understand new situations and ways of working; a willingness to admit when you do not know something; a willingness to ask questions and a desire to increase your understanding and the understanding of others when you are in a position to do so.

When we fail to embrace these key values as individual nurses, or nursing students, it is not only ourselves that we fail, but also the wider team, organisation and ultimately our patients.

Activity 8.5 — Critical thinking

Your orientation to learning environments will influence your understanding and feelings about learning environments. Think about how the environments in the various clinical areas that you have worked in have affected your learning. Consider how you have responded to the various learning opportunities presented to you:

- What have you done when the learning opportunities appear poor?
- Do you ask questions?
- Do you try to supplement this with your own reading and finding out?
- When faced with a poor learning environment do you try to help more junior staff or students with their learning?
- What factors in the ward environment affect the learning opportunities available?
- Can you identify personal or group behaviours which appear to make a difference?

As this is based on your own observations, there is no specimen answer at the end of the chapter.

The questions in this activity point to the role you might play in creating your own learning opportunities regardless of the culture of the place in which you are working. They ask questions about whether you role model positive learning behaviours and take a proactive stance in your own learning and that of others.

You are also asked to reflect on individual and group behaviours which impact on your learning and that of others in the area. Reflecting on and being aware of the behaviours and attitudes that promote, or hinder, learning equips you with ideas about how you might behave in order to promote a positive learning environment. What is important is you realise that issues you have reflected on as a student or junior member of staff become action points for your future career. When you see good practice you might choose to mirror it when you are a leader or manager and when you see poor practice, or practices which do not work very well, you learn from these and do not repeat the same mistakes when you are in a position of influence.

Activity 8.6 — Critical thinking

Given your orientation to learning environments and your experience of them to date, consider how you might go about creating a learning environment in the clinical setting:

- What strategies might you use to promote the change?
- How will you sell the idea to others?
- What strategies for learning might you promote to others?

continued overleaf...

continued... •

The project management template below might help you plan your answer to this activity in a constructive manner.

As this is based on your own observations, there is no specimen answer at the end of the chapter.

Project management template
What is the purpose of the project? What do we do now and what is it we are trying to achieve?
Who is responsible for what aspect of the project? What skills and resources do we have available to us?
Who are our stakeholders? Who will this project affect and how will we get people on board with the idea?
How will we make a start? What do we need to do to start the change process?
What are the possible outcomes, both positive and negative? Consider here personal, team, organisational and patients.
What things might hinder the project and what might help it progress? What are the personnel and financial costs attached?
What should we have achieved by when and how will we know we have achieved these goals?
What will this look like when it is implemented? How will we know we have achieved our ultimate goals?
How and how often will we audit what we have done and maintain impetus assuming we achieve our goals? What measure both direct and indirect might there be of our success?

The purpose of this activity is to demonstrate the thinking, planning, communicating and team working that needs to go into the initiation of a change project. Committing to becoming more learning orientated for yourself and developing a learning culture in a team require commitment, time, effort and good communication. By working through the template you should now be more familiar with the sorts of processes required to make such an important change.

Chapter summary

In this chapter we have seen that environments or cultures of care are important in the functioning of health and social care teams. We have identified that learning cultures are important for the sustained development of nursing teams, and the wider health care system. We have identified that for learning cultures to succeed there is a need for engagement of all of the members of the team. The role of the individual nurse or nursing student within the team has been identified as being fundamental to the success of any culture.

continued opposite...

continued...

The challenge that has been presented in this chapter has been one of engaging in self development as a learner for yourself before considering taking on the extended task of creating a learning environment in your place of work.

Activities: Brief outline answers

Activity 8.1 (page 126)

For the student transiting through an area as part of their training you may see the area as a place of learning while having a feeling of being an outsider. For the permanent staff they may be comfortable with the area and regard it very much as a place of work. Visiting staff, such as physiotherapists and social workers, may see the area as an extension of a bigger area of work. Patients can view an area as somewhere that they are cared for, somewhere they perhaps sleep, eat and follow the activities of living. Visitors can feel the environment is one in which they do not belong and which is somewhere they can at least leave. When working n the community, your place of work is often someone else's home, a place where you are both at work and a visitor, where they are both patient and home owner.

Activity 8.2 (page 128)

When we engage in open conversation about a topic, we become involved. Being involved in something brings a sense of belonging and worth. This sense of worth helps us to understand our place in contributing to something bigger than ourselves, in this case the collective understanding of the topic. This reflects nicely the concept of the learning environment where people feel that they belong because they are not only learning together, they are also contributing to that learning.

Further reading

Clarke, A (2001) *Learning Organisations: What They are and How to Become One.* Leicester: National Institute of Adult Continuing Education.
A comprehensive guide to learning organisations.

Handy, C (1993) *Understanding Organizations.* London: Penguin.
A great and classic text on organisational cultures.

Mullins, LJ (2008) *Essentials of Organisational Behaviour* (2nd edition). London: Prentice Hall.
A comprehensive guide to understanding organisations.

Useful websites

www.nmc-uk.org/Nurses-and-midwives/Advice-by-topic/A/Advice/Environment-of-care
Some guidance on environments of care from the NMC.

www.cipd.co.uk/helpingpeoplelearn/_lrncltre.htm
An interesting selection of case studies about learning cultures from the Chartered Institute of Personnel and Development.

www.pmis.co.uk/free-project-management-templates.htm
A wide collection of interesting and adaptable project templates.

www.investorsinpeople.co.uk/About/PolicyDevelopment/Pages/Engagingemployees.aspx
A useful website about strategies for employee engagement and people development, this page has a link to the report 'Employee Engagement' which is a good primer for any aspiring leader of people.

Chapter 9
Developing confidence as a manager and leader

NMC Standards for Pre-registration Nursing Education

This chapter will address the following competencies:

Domain 1: Professional values

5. All nurses must fully understand the nurse's various roles, responsibilities and functions, and adapt their practice to meet the changing needs of people, groups, communities and populations.

8. All nurses must practise independently, recognising the limits of their competence and knowledge. They must reflect on these limits and seek advice from, or refer to, other professionals where necessary.

Domain 4: Leadership, management and team working

1. All nurses must act as change agents and provide leadership through quality improvement and service development to enhance people's well-being and experiences of healthcare.

3. All nurses must be able to identify priorities and manage time and resources effectively to ensure the quality of care is maintained or enhanced.

Essential Skills Clusters

This chapter will address the following ESCs:

Cluster: Organisational aspects of care

12. People can trust the newly registered graduate nurse to respond to their feedback and a wide range of other sources to learn, develop and improve services.

    At entry to the register:

    8. As an individual team member and team leader, actively seeks and learns from feedback to enhance care and own and others professional development.

16. People can trust the newly registered graduate nurse to safely lead, co-ordinate and manage care.

    At entry to the register:

    1. Inspires confidence and provides clear direction to others.

    3. Bases decisions on evidence and uses experience to guide decision-making.

    4. Acts as a positive role model for others.

> **Chapter aims**
>
> After reading this chapter you will be able to:
>
> - discuss the practice-leadership continuum;
> - demonstrate an awareness of some of the issues with transition to leadership and management roles;
> - discuss some of the key challenges which face new leaders and managers;
> - explain how confidence might be developed in the new manager.

Introduction

Throughout this book we have introduced you to ideas and theories about leadership and management and some of the tasks that leaders and managers undertake; you may have formed the impression there is a lot to learn, and indeed there is. You will also have noted many of the tasks of management start with understanding yourself and your orientation to a situation, role or task. Clearly understanding yourself and being aware of your strengths and weaknesses is as important for succeeding as a leader or manager as it is for nursing in general.

This chapter will look at some of the issues facing the new leader or manager and identify and focus on some strategies that might be used to help develop ability and confidence. Other issues which commonly confront the new manager will also be addressed with some ideas about how these might be handled both proactively and reactively. As with all of the chapters in this book it is important that you engage with the activities presented as they represent tools for self development which may help to enhance both your learning and your development as a manager as well as your confidence to lead.

The transition to leadership

When you first thought about being a nurse and when you were interviewed for your nurse training, it is likely you thought and talked about all of the ways you could help people as a practising nurse. As you progress through your training and into your nursing career you may start to aspire to leadership and management and start to see this as a way of extending the scope of what you can do for and with patients.

It is worth reflecting here on the different stages of professional life we adopt as we move from practising nurse through to leadership and management roles. Causer and Exworthy (2003) identify six stages on the path from practice to management which they regard as being stages on a continuum of roles which health and social care professionals may find themselves on.

> 1. **The Practising Professional**: The main task of the practising professional is the provision of care. Within this definition there are two groups of people:
>
> *continued overleaf...*

continued...

(a) the pure practitioner – who undertakes professional roles but has no supervisory role;

(b) the quasi-managerial practitioner – who undertakes a professional caring role, and has some responsibility for supervising others or allocating resources.

2. **The Managing Professional**: The main function of these professionally trained managers is the supervision of other professionals and the allocation and management of resources. Again this group is split into two groups:

(a) the practising managing professional – who still works in the delivery of care as well as managing others and resources;

(b) the non-practising managing professional – who does not deliver care, but supervises other professionals and manages resources.

3. **General Managers**: Managers who manage others who are involved in the delivery of professional care, but not at the day-to-day (**operational**) level. Again these are subdivided into two categories:

(a) non-professionally grounded general managers – who are not part of the profession they are managing;

(b) professionally grounded general managers – who are part of the profession they are managing.

Roles within the professional-management continuum
Source: Adapted from Causer and Exworthy, (2003)

What Causer and Exworthy (2003) identify is that the transition from being a practitioner to being a manager can be one which is subtle and takes place over a series of stages. The move from practice to management is therefore not a stark one whereby one day you are a nurse practising on the ward and the next day you are a general manager far removed from the realities of day-to-day care. The process identified here will most certainly allow for some adaptation and personal and professional development to take place. This notion links well with the ideas around being a learning organisation and individual identified in Chapter 8.

Activity 9.1   *Critical thinking*

Taking the categories of professionals and managers that Causer and Exworthy identify, consider all of the people who work in the team in the clinical area in which you are, or were last, placed. Which of the roles identified in the model do they fit into, if any? What characteristics of Causer and Exworthy's descriptions do they display? What was their previous role? You may want to take this activity a step further and discuss the changing nature of the individual's roles with them.

As this is based on your own observations, there is no specimen answer at the end of the chapter.

Undertaking this activity will help you to discover that there are layers of responsibility, leadership and management in the clinical setting. The degree of certainty people have in the roles they undertake can grow and develop as they move from one position to another within the team, or between teams, and as they learn from their own practice and from those around them. What is important in the transition from practice to management remains the focus on the values which you came into nursing with (see Chapter 1) and a willingness to develop both yourself and others around you (see Chapter 8).

Self esteem and transition

As with all development, the changes which need to occur for you to move from school, or from another job, to becoming a nursing student, to qualifying and beyond, require some psychological adjustment. Even when we are excited about something there are adjustments to make to the ways in which we think and behave as we move on to something new. Sometimes the adjustments we have to make are in response to whatever it was we aspired to not quite living up to what we expected from it. Either way, it is worth considering the nature of change and transition from being a practising nurse to being a leader.

Activity 9.2   *Reflection*

Consider some time in your life when you have had to make adjustments to accommodate a change which you wanted to make. How did you feel? What emotions did you experience? Now think about a change you had not planned for and did not want to make. How did you feel? What emotions did you experience? Were there emotions or feelings which were common to both scenarios?

There are some possible answers and thoughts at the end of the chapter.

Some of your answers to the above reflection will show the emotions experienced during a change are similar regardless of whether it was planned or not. What this tells us for planning to make the change from practitioner to leader or manager is there are a host of normal emotions and responses to change we need to prepare for.

Perhaps the first lesson is that an emotional response to change is normal and is not something we should be shy or embarrassed about. This applies even if the change is something we want and are looking forward to. You should therefore not be surprised if you are a little stressed by a promotion or when you are given a leadership role; it is normal!

It is worth stopping again here and considering the nature of the emotional responses that people have as they adapt and evolve.

Bridges (2003), a leading thinker and writer about the change process, reminds us that things change, but people go through transitions. A fundamental tenet of Bridges' position is that transition involves loss and letting go, as well as developing a new understanding of how things are. In the case of the nurse making the transition from practising nurse to leader or manager, this involves a redefining of her professional and personal identity. Bridges' model of transition captures these ideas in a three stage process.

---

1. **Ending, Losing, Letting Go**: At this stage people have to make the adjustment to not being who they were before. For example, a student nurse on the point of

continued overleaf...

continued...

qualifying must adjust to being a qualified and accountable nurse; or a staff nurse being promoted to being a junior sister may have to adapt to being more visible to others and the hub of questions and responsibility.

2. **The Neutral Zone**: At this stage people try to make sense of who they are now and how things are going to be. Student nurses start to accept they are now qualified and begin to adopt the persona of someone who is accountable for what they are doing; junior charge nurses start to understand they have to be the one to find solutions to problems and act as a role model to the team.

3. **The New Beginning**: A new identify is forming and there is increased clarity about what is expected in the new role. There is a sense of urgency and of wanting to get on with the job. New staff nurses start to feel confident in their own ability and what they are doing; the new sister or charge nurse feels comfortable about being a role model and overseeing the work of the team.

Three-phase process of transition (adapted from Bridges, 2003).

While progressing through the process of changing identity, what we have called transition, it is normal for people to experience a whole range of different emotions. These emotions, as we discussed earlier, can arise even if the change is something that is wanted. Understanding these emotions and recognising them in yourself, as well as others, is a good way of helping maintain and develop your confidence as you progress through your nursing career.

Hopson and Adams (1976) propose a useful, and enduring, model which helps identify some of the stages people go through when they are subject to transition. This model, presented below, is not a linear one (people move through it in different directions at different rates and may skip stages), nor does it necessarily apply to all transitions people go through; nevertheless, it is a useful model for helping us to understand the emotional response to transition.

Immobilisation: The feeling of being unable to act and overwhelmed because of a transition. Transitions for which people are unprepared and ones associated with negative expectations may intensify this stage.

Minimisation: A coping mechanism. People often deny the change is happening. This reaction is common in a crisis which is too difficult to face head-on.

Depression: Some people become depressed when they have to face the reality of change.

Accepting Reality: Occurs when a person going through a transition begins to let go of how things were and starts to accept the reality of the change.

Testing: Begins when the reality of the change has been accepted. At this stage people start to try out new behaviours to cope with the new situation.

Seeking meaning: A reflective stage during which people try to work out how and why things are different.

continued opposite...

continued...

Internalisation: The final stage of the process during which the new situation becomes accepted. The new understanding then becomes part of the person's behaviour.

Changes in self-esteem during transitions
Source: Adapted from Hopson and Adams (1976)

When making the transition from student nurse to trained nurse and then on to leader and manager it is useful for us to be aware of the ways in which we react to change as individuals. Being aware of our own responses enables us to make sense of and progress through the various stages of emotional response to change as well as managing how we behave around and towards other people.

Being aware of the range of emotions experienced during times of transition also allows us to provide appropriate support to staff during periods of change and transition in their lives. Change and transition is not only confined to the workplace: changes in home circumstances, bereavement, ill health, etc. will all impact on how managers and their staff feel and behave. Being aware of this and maintaining good channels of communication will allow the leader or manager to develop skills and confidence in people management which are closely associated with emotional intelligence.

Activity 9.3 — *Critical thinking*

Now that you have seen Hopson and Adams' model of the changes in self esteem during change, can you relate to any of the stages identified for yourself, or in others? Now that you understand something more of the ways in which people respond to transition, what strategies do you think you can employ as an individual or as a leader to help people adjust to change?

There are some possible answers and thoughts at the end of the chapter.

Clearly, being prepared for the emotional response which you may have to a change in your role or work circumstances means you will be able to reflect on what is happening and better prepare yourself mentally for the challenges ahead. As a leader or manager, providing support to your team through supervision, information giving and being generally supportive will mean you can help reduce some of the impact of negative emotional responses to transition.

Activity 9.4 — *Evidence-based practice and research*

To better understand the nature of the emotional responses to change people have, look up the **Holmes-Rahe Life Event Rating Scale** and read the categories of change that people find most stressful in their lives; some of the listed changes may surprise you.

As this is based on your own observations, there is no specimen answer at the end of the chapter.

Having a growing understanding of your own responses to change will enable you to face the transitions required to progress throughout your career in nursing with a renewed degree of confidence. Preparing yourself mentally and emotionally for the impact of transition will mean you are better prepared for some of the challenges of leadership and management.

Developing yourself as a leader

The purpose of this book has been to prepare you for some of the challenges being a leader or manager can present. This section of the book will present and examine some of the strategies you can use to better prepare yourself for a leadership or management role whilst being aware of, and managing, your own emotional response to change. All of the ideas presented here are tools and tactics that can be used while a student or junior staff nurse in order to improve and enhance your own confidence, better understand yourself and develop some self discipline in your approach to managing yourself.

Williams (2007, page 51) tells us: 'exceptional leaders have the ability to honestly assess their leadership skills – and the discipline to improve their weaknesses and build upon their strengths'. Only you can truly know whether you are willing to put effort into your self-development.

Set incremental goals

Target setting is a key factor in self motivation. If you cannot be bothered to write an essay or to complete an application form then whatever it is you are aiming to do will not happen. Motivation is an interesting tool both in personal and professional development as well as from the point of view of the leader or manager. Herzberg (1959), the most enduring and famous theorist in this area, proposed the Motivation-Hygiene Theory of job satisfaction. In essence, Herzberg's theory suggests that people will work hard in order to achieve the hygiene needs as without them they are unhappy. Once the hygiene factors are achieved people are happy, but only for a short time. It is only the true motivators which keep people happy and motivate them and offer a true sense of meaning for individuals.

Hygiene factors

- quality of relationships with supervisors
- working conditions
- salary
- status
- job security
- quality of relationship with subordinates
- personal life

True motivators

- achievement
- recognition

continued opposite...

continued...

- opportunity for advancement
- work itself
- responsibility
- sense of personal growth

Motivation-hygiene theory of job satisfaction

Source: Aadapted from Herzberg (1959)

What we can see both for ourselves and for others is that motivation lies in taking responsibility and improving on what we do and therefore who we are. For the student this may mean getting better at writing essays, by learning from feedback to achieve better marks and hence recognition. For the leader it may be important to ensure the hygiene factors are all in place before worrying too much about the motivators.

Case study: Recognising the value of motivation

Jacinta had recently been promoted to Modern Matron in the surgical care team. Jacinta had worked her way up through the team over a period of years and was very much aware of the issues which preoccupied the staff. She knew that staff morale was very low as the team felt overworked, understaffed, poorly cared for and generally neglected. Jacinta understood the team felt the need for further professional development as well as some clarity about promotion opportunities. Jacinta was also aware that the whole team were fed up with the state of their coffee room, which had been allowed to deteriorate over time. She knew she needed to do something quick to raise the morale of the whole team and to consolidate her position as the team leader but she also knew she had limited funds with which to do anything.

Jacinta considered her options and decided there were some things she could do collectively for the team as well as some things she needed to do for individuals within the team in order to raise morale, gain trust and improve motivation. Jacinta decided to spend some of the capital budget available to her to buy new furniture for the coffee room. By doing so she improved working conditions for the whole team and addressed a hygiene need.

Jacinta quickly realised she could not provide the motivation the staff needed purely by spending money (which was not available to her anyway) so she identified new roles for various members of the team as link nurses for infection control, diabetes and wound management, providing some of the junior staff with a sense of increased responsibility, recognition and personal growth. Furthermore, Jacinta took it upon herself to try to make sure staff went home when their shifts ended. She praised effort and cultivated her relationships within the team, addressing key hygiene and motivational needs.

This case study, which is based on a real life experience, demonstrates how easy it can be to grow as a leader or manager in the eyes of the team by making small but important changes. Facilitating and bringing about the changes meant that not only did the team feel happier, but Jacinta's confidence as a manager grew as she started to notice a change in the morale of the team and that the team had started to trust her as someone who both cared about them and was able to get things done.

Learn to listen

For the nurse as much as the leader or manager, listening is a fundamental skill. When we learn to listen to others, be it in a formal context or by listening to informal sources of information, then we can understand the true context of situations. Listening also enables us to find solutions to problems which we may not have identified for ourselves.

Listening is a key skill for the leader or manager in understanding what the team are thinking and what is important to them. Managing information was identified in Chapter 6 as one of Mintzberg's (1975) roles of the manager. Information allows us to make decisions which are well grounded and learning to listen and to be enquiring will enhance your ability both to understand what is going on around you and to make sound decisions.

In this context listening is more about taking the time to hear what people are saying and trying to understand it while placing what we are hearing in the context of what we know. As an active skill, listening is important for personal growth and for professional development within healthcare which is a complex and evolving environment within which to work (Jackson and Ellis, 2010). For the developing leader listening means you can be confident you understand what is going on around you.

Understand then communicate

The ultimate aim of listening properly and effectively is to understand. Understanding situations and new ideas is a good way of developing your confidence. Part of understanding is the ability to ask the right questions at the right time as well as being able to communicate your ideas in an effective way. Communicating effectively hinges on your ability to understand what other people know as well as what it is they want.

As a leader or manager your confidence will develop as people become aware that you are able to communicate clearly. Clear communication will mean members of the team understand what it is you want from them, it allows you to delegate effectively and explain ideas. Learning to think and understand before speaking is a key skill for the aspiring leader or manager; we have all been in situations when individuals have made themselves look silly because they have said something or asked a question which clearly demonstrates they have not been listening; being thought of as silly is not a good place to be for the new leader or manager!

Believe in yourself

Self belief is not the same as arrogance or being egocentric. Self belief is having the confidence you can do something well and doing it. Self belief comes only from practice, from exercising your leadership muscles by developing and maintaining good relationships with staff and understanding yourself. When you believe in what you are doing as well as believing you have the ability to do it, other people will see this self belief and feel able to follow your lead.

Leaders and managers who are confident in their own abilities are better able to develop their team and are comfortable with members of the team having better skills and knowledge in certain areas than they do. The manager who has self belief will recognise that the team is more important than self and this team focused attitude will help develop trust within the team.

Don't be afraid to make mistakes

Making mistakes is part of life. This is as true for the leader or manager as it is for individual team workers. Learning to reflect enables us to make sense of what has happened as well as learning how to do something better in the future (see Reflective Practice in Nursing, also in this series). Learning from our mistakes can make us stronger as individuals and as leaders as we develop new ways of working which take account of what we have learnt as well as where we want to be. Failure often precedes success as it is through trying new ways of working that we are able to be innovative (Farson and Keyes, 2002).

Part of the process of growing as a person and a leader is the ability to accept responsibility for the things we get wrong. When, as leaders, we develop the ability to accept responsibility for our own actions we can role model responsibility and accountability to our team.

Within the team context supporting others who make mistakes empowers them to make decisions and take actions with the confidence they will be supported; again this is a key element of trust. SanFacon (2008) reminds leaders that in order to achieve success they need to trust in their staff and allow them to make mistakes. So being brave enough to try new things and new ways of working is useful in developing your confidence in yourself and in your ability to lead others.

Learn to manage your time effectively

As a leader or manager the way in which you use time is important. The pressures on time as a leader of people come in all shapes and forms and can quite easily disrupt your working day. Time management is the art of getting the most from your time by developing an awareness of what time is and how it is used. Understanding the importance of time and how to use it wisely will help you understand what you can achieve and in what time frame. This will translate into the confidence to take on new roles and tasks or allow you to explain why you cannot.

John Adair (1990), whose model of action centred leadership we looked at in Chapter 6, suggests leaders and managers need to learn to manage time before they can manage anything else. In Adair's view good time management is a requirement for allowing us to focus on what we do and achieve our goals. Time management is therefore about being focused on attaining our goals and achieving results and in Adair's view there are ten principles by which good time management can be achieved by a leader or manager.

> **Theory summary: Adair's ten principles of good time management**
>
> 1. **Develop a personal sense of time:** this is about understanding where your time goes and therefore understanding where it is wasted and where it could be better used. For the leader it may also uncover areas of work which might be better delegated to someone else.
>
> *continued overleaf...*

continued...

2. **Identify long-term goals:** this is about knowing what it is you want to achieve in life and work. Adair recognises values as being a key driving force behind setting such goals.

3. **Make medium-term plans:** understand what things you need to do in order to prepare you to achieve your long-term goals and plan what you need to do now to achieve them. Medium-term plans involve setting realistic goals which are measurable.

4. **Plan the day:** without planning what you will achieve today, you cannot know whether you have used your time wisely at the end of the day. Learning to say no to things which are a poor use of your time or which interfere with you achieving your goals is important here.

5. **Make the best use of your best time:** understand what times of day you work best and work during them. Take time to think about issues and ideas which need planning while doing other more mundane activities.

6. **Organise office work:** make sure that you organise your life and your working space so things you need are at hand when you need them.

7. **Manage meetings:** understand what you want from a meeting or other period of communication with other people and stick to the time available for this.

8. **Delegate effectively:** consider what things you need to do and what might be better done by someone else.

9. **Make use of committed time:** plan to use time that is usually wasted waiting or travelling and be prepared to use this to good effect, perhaps reading something, making phone calls or thinking constructively about an issue.

10. **Manage your health:** things are easier to achieve when we are well so look after yourself and make time to do things necessary for your physical and mental well-being.

Source: Adapted from Adair (1990).

For Adair, understanding and being aware of time and how we use it is key to personal success. Making good use of time and being aware of what we can achieve in a given time frame are key to developing confidence in ourselves both as individuals and as leaders or managers. When you know what you achieved and why it is a great motivator.

Activity 9.5 — *Evidence-based practice and research*

Keep a diary of all the things you do for one week. Split the time into 15 minute slots and record what you do and be careful to record wasted time as well as activities. After one week review the diary and identify times during which you could have done something useful if you were prepared. Consider how you might adapt some of your ways of working and habits to allow you to achieve more in the time available to you. You may wish to use this exercise as a springboard for planning your personal development and planning what you want to achieve, how and by when. Understanding how you use time will enable you to plan this more effectively.

As this is based on your own observations, there is no specimen answer at the end of the chapter.

Once you understand how you use time and where you can fit in tasks to make your use of time more efficient you will start to see that it is possible to fit more into your day. When you free up time you can decide how you are going to use it, perhaps undertaking more work or engaging in a hobby or other interest.

Know your values

You may feel that we have discussed values too much in this book; however, since our values shape the ways we behave their importance cannot be overestimated. Knowing what your values are as a human, as a nurse and ultimately as a leader or manager will mean there is some consistency in the ways in which you act. Sticking to your values will not only mean you are happier in whatever you do, it will mean the team will know what to expect from you and, perhaps more importantly, what you expect from them. In part trust, which is the means by which leaders get things done, relies on leaders demonstrating their integrity to their followers (Lawton, 1998).

One of the issues which face nurses as they move from practice to leadership and management roles is their lack of clarity about their identity. It is easy to forget the things which mattered to you as a student or staff nurse, the values which guided your desire to be a nurse and your subsequent practice as you become more engaged with leadership and management roles. Understanding what your values are now and being able to discuss them in a meaningful way will help you remain grounded and focused as you prepare for leadership.

Activity 9.6   *Reflection*

Take some time now to consider the things which you value as a human being and as a nurse. Think about the things you might have said at interview about why you wanted to train as a nurse or the skills and attributes which you bring to your current role. Consider the issues in practice which cause you frustration and the behaviours which you think are unacceptable from your colleagues. Write these things down and keep them safe. Spend some time over the next few weeks thinking and observing these issues in practice and considering what you might do to change poor practice and role model good leadership values when you are in a position to do so.

As this is based on your own observations, there is no specimen answer at the end of the chapter.

Issues such as fairness, treating people as equals, being polite and treating people with care and compassion might feature on your list. These are all basic values which are easily forgotten in the milieu of the busy working day. Practising these values and ensuring they become part of who you are and how you act will allow you to establish a reputation not only as someone who knows what they are doing but also as someone who knows who they are and what they are about.

Develop resilience

One of the hallmarks of the strong leader or manager is the ability to be resilient. Resilience is the ability to take criticism constructively, listen to what people are saying about your organisation and team without taking it personally and the ability to understand the meaning of situations.

Resilience is not all about developing a thick skin, not least of all because a thick skin prevents effective empathy. Resilience is more about having the ability to deal with stressful situations. It is important here again to understand yourself. If you understand what things you find stressful and why, you can learn to manage them.

Case study: Developing resilience

Mee-Onn was a newly appointed junior sister on a general medical ward. She had come from a different hospital to take on the new role and did not know any of the team. Mee-Onn found that the staff and the patients on the ward were very free and easy about making complaints, grumbling and suggesting how things might be done better.

As the junior sister, Mee-Onn was often the target of these suggestions and gripes. Mee-Onn found it hard to cope with all of the information and after a few weeks in post started to take all of the negative comments personally, as if they were a reflection on her. She started to feel very stressed and did not want to go to work any more. Mee-Onn discussed her feelings with the medical matron. The matron, who had come up through the ranks in the hospital, suggested to Mee-Onn that she stopped taking all of the criticism as personal and that she turned issues back to the staff with questions like 'how would you see this progressing?' or 'what would you suggest we do to improve this?' The matron also suggested Mee-Onn did not accept some of the unfair things people were saying and that she should tell them what they were saying was unfair.

Asking these simple questions reminded Mee-Onn that the problems were not hers alone. She developed the strength to confront some of the situations and issues which plagued the team and started to be seen as someone with solutions. She also developed a reputation for being fair-minded and not someone who would tolerate unreasonable behaviour.

This study, again based on a real life story, demonstrates that one of the skills of being a leader or manager is learning what a gripe or moan means and who it is aimed at. It also demonstrates how taking on board issues which are not personal, and are not purely your own problem, may lead to a sense of helplessness and futility. Taking charge of such situations by being brave enough to ask for a solution, rather than saying something like 'I know what you mean', can help you as the leader develop delegation skills and demonstrate trust. It can also help you move away from being weak and downtrodden.

So in part resilience is about developing strategies to deflect and reflect problems back to where they really belong; of course this does not mean every problem which comes your way!

Confront challenging situations

Developing resilience leads us nicely into the next skill which is about not being afraid to get involved. There are times as a nurse that situations arise and people behave in ways which we feel are less than acceptable. Such situations need confronting and learning to communicate your point in a way which links in with your express values is a good place to start. Certainly as a manager or leader there is nowhere to hide and learning to confront difficult situations early is a good idea. One strategy for the novice is to accompany more experienced staff who are, for example, breaking bad news, ask questions about what they did after the event and reflect on the answers.

The other sort of challenging situation is one which you do not understand or about which you are uncertain. The key to developing the ability to confront such a situation is developing the ability to ask questions. Asking questions allows for understanding and should not be mistaken for weakness. As an aspiring leader it is important you develop a reputation for being enquiring and that you support others in their efforts to achieve self awareness and self development.

Develop your emotional intelligence

Perhaps many of the messages which are contained in this book can be boiled down to one key message: develop your emotional intelligence. Throughout the book we have suggested there is a need to understand yourself and the part you play in many situations before you look at what other people are doing or saying. You also need to understand where other people are coming from and what motivates their actions.

Emotional intelligence requires you to be able to use this understanding of the emotional motivation which you and other people have in order to communicate effectively. Emotional intelligence and awareness of motivations as well as the ability and desire to help others achieve their goals reflect strongly on many of the standards of proficiency and essential skills highlighted at the start of this chapter.

Activity 9.7 *Reflection*

Consider the standards of proficiency and essential skill clusters identified at the start of the chapter and how these relate to the ability of the individual nurse to understand themselves and others. Reflect on how being emotionally literate will enable you to achieve many of the standards and skills identified and what you will do in order to demonstrate you have the necessary skills and values in place to achieve them.

As this is based on your own reflections, there is no specimen answer at the end of the chapter.

You will notice many of the skills, attributes and roles which nurses undertake require them to be self aware and aware of the needs of others. This awareness, which you are required to develop as a student nurse, will most certainly be a big part of the suite of skill competencies which we have suggested in this book go towards creating effective managers and leaders. What is important for you as you develop from student nurse to staff nurse, sister and beyond is that you conscientiously continue to develop these capabilities in such a way that they become part of who you are and therefore how you behave. Nurse leaders and managers are entrusted with the management and leadership of people delivering care to some of the most vulnerable in society. By becoming a good role model you can be more certain the care you and your team deliver lives up to the lofty ideals of modern nursing practice.

Chapter summary

In this chapter we have explored the journey from student nurse to nurse manager and what this might mean for us in managing our emotional responses to change and transition. We

continued overleaf...

• *continued...* •

have identified a number of important strategies, skills, tactics and values which taken together can better prepare you for the responsibilities that leadership and management bring.

We have identified that the core values and skills of nursing translate well into leadership and management roles and hence the need for student nurses and junior staff nurses to develop, practise and hone these skills from an early point in their career.

Activities: Brief outline answers

Activity 9.2 (page 139)

The sorts of emotions that people feel as they experience different changes and transitions in their lives are not purely tied to the sort of change they are experiencing. All change can bring fear and trepidation, even the changes that are wanted and exciting. Underestimating the impact of transition on yourself or on others will mean that you are ill-prepared to understand your own responses and provide support to others.

Activity 9.3 (page 141)

Being aware of people's responses to change will mean you are prepared for and can understand the emotions you experience as you go through transitions for yourself. You will also be able to identify and provide support for staff and colleagues subject to change by responding appropriately to their needs as they progress through the transition. Failure to recognise that someone is depressed or seeking new meaning may mean as a leader or manager we misinterpret their behaviours and perhaps treat them in a less than supportive manner.

Further reading

Bennis, WG (2004) The Seven Ages of the Leader. *Harvard Business Review*, 82 (1): 46–53.
An inspiring and informational look at leadership development.

Davis, N. (2011) *Learning Skills for Nursing Students.* Exeter: Learning Matters.
Gives helpful advice for gaining knowledge and confidence.

Useful websites

www.businessballs.com/self-confidence-assertiveness.htm
A useful and interesting take on developing self confidence.

http://labspace.open.ac.uk/mod/resource/view.php?id=369014
A quick overview of Hopson and Adams' model of self esteem during transition.

**http://changingminds.org/disciplines/change_management/psychology_change/
psychology_change.htm**
A quirky but informative look at the psychology of change and transition.

www.learnmanagement2.com/managementconcepts.htm
Some good pages on motivational theories can be found here.

www.cipd.co.uk/subjects/lrnanddev/selfdev/emotintel.htm?IsSrchRes=1
The Chartered Institute of Personnel and Development's synopsis of emotional intelligence.

Glossary

binary thinking in the sense used here it refers to a way of defining your identity with reference to the differences between you and someone else.

clinical supervision a process of guided group reflection facilitated by a third party.

emotional intelligence being aware of your own emotions, the emotions in others and how these modify behaviours and being able to talk about this in a meaningful way with others.

Gantt chart the most common format for displaying project outlines and progress. Named after Henry Gantt, who developed it in the early 1900s, the chart is a form of bar chart which displays activities or events plotted against time.

governance the methods by which organisations follow regulations stipulated by higher governing bodies to ensure standards are met through their authoritative structures.

group think a phenomenon that occurs when the members of a group make a collective decision based on seeking unanimity rather than encouraging individual reasoning or critical evaluation of ideas.

Hawthorne effect changes which occur in people's behaviour because they know they are being observed.

Holmes-Rahe Life Event Rating Scale a scale of 43 life events which are scored by the amount of stress they can cause. A high score means more stress. Some of the changes are positive ones but still cause significant stress.

integrity staying true to your own moral and ethical principles.

learning cultures/organisations/teams groups of people who learn from, and with, each other in the workplace and use this learning to enhance what they do.

legitimate power the power to lead and manage that an individual has by virtue of their position within an organisation as well as their ability to use that power in a reasonable, perhaps ethical, manner.

mediation resolution of conflict through the facilitation of an impartial third party.

negotiation/negotiate the process of reaching a compromise agreement through talking.

operational referring to the management of the day-to-day tasks of an organisation or team.

othering the process whereby anyone who does not share the same characteristics as us is seen to be 'other'. If we are nurses, non-nurses are 'other'.

outcomes in the sense they are used in this book, outcomes refer not only to the result of a care episode but also the individual's experience of care. Quality is therefore seen as achieving health goals as well as providing health care in a manner acceptable to and involving the client.

person-centred referring to care which is provided with the needs and wants of the patients at its core. This is the opposite of providing care which is dictated by what health and social care professionals want to provide or which is rigidly dictated by policy.

skill mix an appropriate number of people of various levels of ability on duty at the same time in order to be able to undertake the tasks required during a shift.

social capital building up a bank of good will that can be called on later when you need a favour or support.

span of control the number of employees for which each organisation manager or head of department is responsible.

stakeholders individuals who will be affected directly or indirectly as a result of the organisation's actions, objectives, outcomes.

total quality management an approach to quality management that takes account of both the outcome of the care episode and the ways in which the care episode was experienced by the patient or client.

values the personal rules and understandings we have about what is right and what is wrong in human behaviour.

whistle blowing the process of raising the alarm about some poor practice usually through an established channel.

References

Adair, J (1990) *How to Manage your Time*. Guildford: Talbot Adair Press.

Adair, J (2010) *Develop your Leadership Skills*. London: Kogan Page.

Aiken, LH, Clarke, SP, Sloane, DL, Sochalski, J and Silber, JH (2002) Hospital Nurse Staffing and Patient Mortality, Nurse Burnout and Job Dissatisfaction. *Journal of American Medical Association*, 23/30, 288 (16): 1987–93.

Anderson, RA, Corazzini, KN and McDaniel, RR (2004) Complexity Science and the Dynamics of Climate and Communication: Reducing Nursing Home Turnover. *The Gerontologist*, 44: 378–88.

Antai-Otong, D (1997) *Team Building in a Health Care Setting. American Journal of Nursing*, 97 (7): 48–51.

Bach, S and Grant, A (2011) *Communication and Interpersonal Skills for Nurses* (2nd edition). Exeter: Learning Matters.

Barrack, MR and Mount, MK (1991) The Big Five Personality Dimensions and Job Performance: A Meta Analysis. *Personnel Psychology*, 44 (41): 1–26.

Bass, BM (1985) *Leadership and Performance*. New York: Free Press.

Beckhard, RF and Harris, RT (1987) *Organisation Transitions: Managing Complex Change*. Boston: Addison Wesley.

Belbin, MR (2010) *Management Teams: Why They Succeed or Fail* (3rd edition). Oxford: Butterworth Heinemann.

Bennis, WG (1989) *On Becoming a Leader*. New York: Addison Wesley.

Bersin, J (2010) Create a High-Impact Learning Culture. *Chief Learning Officer*, 9 (10): 16.

Bondas, T (2006) Paths to Nursing Leadership. *Journal of Nursing Management*, 14: 332–9.

Bray, L and Nettleton, P (2007) Assessor or Mentor? Role Confusion in Professional Education. *Nurse Education Today*, 27 (8): 848–55.

Bridges, W (2003) *Managing Transitions: Making the Most of Change*. London: Nicholas Brearley.

Bullman, A, Charlesworth, J, Henderson, J, Reynolds, J and Seden, J (2003) (eds) *The Managing Care Reader*. London: Routledge.

Butterworth, T, Bell, L, Jackson, C and Majda, P (2007) Wicked Spell or Magic Bullet? A Review of the Clinical Supervision Literature 2001–2007. *Nurse Education Today*, 28 (3): 24–272.

Care Quality Commission (2011) *Care Quality Commission demands action after report identifies failings at Cambridgeshire and Peterborough NHS Trust*. Available online at: www.cqc.org.uk/newsandevents/ pressreleases.cfm?cit_id=37178&FAArea1=customWidgets.content_view_1&usecache=false (accessed May 2011).

Causer, G and Exworthy, M (2003) Professionals as Managers Across the Public Sector, in Bullman, A, Charlesworth, J, Henderson, J, Reynolds, J and Seden, J (eds) *The Managing Care Reader* (pages 213–19). London: Routledge.

Chartered Institute of Personnel and Development (2007) *Managing Conflict at Work*: Survey Report. London: CIPD.

Chartered Institute of Personnel and Development (2011) *Performance Appraisal Factsheet*. Available online at: www.cipd.co.uk/hr-resources/factsheets/performance-appraisal.aspx (accessed April 2011).

Clews, G (2010) *Lack of Support for Nurses Blamed for Mid Staffs Failings*. Available online at: www.nursingtimes.net/whats-new-in-nursing/acute-care/lack-of-support-for-nurses-blamed-for-mid-staffs-failings/5011861.article (accessed 12 October 2010).

Croskerry, P and Norman, G (2008) Overconfidence in Clinical Decision Making. *American Journal of Medicine*, 121: S24–S29.

Cummings, G and McLennan, M (2005) Advanced Practice Nursing. Leadership to effect policy change. *Journal of Nursing Administration*, 35 (2): 61–6.

Daft, R (2001) *The Leadership Experience* (2nd edition). Florence, Kentucky: South-Western Educational Publishing.

Darzi, A. (2008) *High-Quality Care For All: NHS Next Stage Review final report*. London: Department of Health.

Davies, C (2004) Workers, Professions and Identity, in Henderson, J and Atkinson, D (eds) *Managing Care in Context* (pages189–210). London: Routledge.

Davis, N (2011) *Learning Skills for Nursing Students*. Exeter: Learning Matters.

Dawson, A and Butler, I (2004) The Morally Active Manager, in Henderson, J and Atkinson, D (eds) *Managing Care in Context* (papers 237–58). London: Routledge.

Dawson and Butler (2004)

Deakins, D and Freel, M (2009) *Entrepreneurship and Small Firms* (5th edition). London: McGraw Hill.

Drennan, V, Davis, K, Traynor, M, Goodman, C, Mark, A, Peacock, R, Humphrey, C and Fairley-Murray, S (2007) Entrepreneurial Nurses and Midwives in the United Kingdom: An Integrative Review. *Journal of Advanced Nursing*, 60 (5): 459–69.

Edwards, D, Burnard, P, Hannigan, B, Cooper, L, Adams, J, Juggessur, T, Fothergil, A and Coyle, D (2006) Clinical Supervision and Burnout: The Influence of Clinical Supervision for Community Mental Health Nurses. *Journal of Clinical Nursing*, 15: 1007–10.

Ellis, P (2010) *Understanding Research for Nursing Students (Transforming Nursing Practice)*. Exeter: Learning Matters.

Ellis, P and Abbott, J (2010) How to Learn to Delegate Effectively in the Renal Unit. *Journal of Renal Nursing*, 2 (2): 38–40.

Farson, R and Keyes, R (2002) The Failure Tolerant Leader. *Harvard Business Review*, 80 (8): 64–71.

Fowler, A (1996) How to Provide Effective Feedback. *People Management*, 2 (14): 44–5.

Frankel, A (2008) What Leadership Styles should Senior Nurses Develop? *Nursing Times*, 104 (35): 23–4.

French, JPR Jr and Raven, B (1960) The Bases of Social Power, in Cartwright D and Zander, A (eds) *Group Dynamics* (pages 607–23). New York: Harper and Row.

Gainsborough, S (2009) Risks and Benefits: Changing the Nursing Skill Mix. *Nursing Times*, 22 (September). Available online at: www.nursingtimes.net/whats-new-in-nursing/acute-care/risks-and-benefits-changing-the-nursing-skill-mix/5006399.article.

Gallway, T (1974) *The Inner Game of Tennis*. New York: Random House.

Gallway, T (2000) *The Inner Game of Work*. New York: Random House.

Gantt, HL (1910) Work, Wages and Profit, published by *The Engineering Magazine*, New York; republished as *Work, Wages and Profits*, Easton, PA: Hive Publishing Company, 1974.

Goleman, D (1996) *Emotional Intelligence: Why it can Matter more than IQ*. London: Bloomsbury.

Goleman, D (1998) *Working with Emotional Intelligence*. New York: Bantam Books.

Goodwin, B and Clemow, R (2010) *Nursing and Interprofessional Practice* (2nd edition). Exeter: Learning Matters.

Grant, AM (2001) *Towards a Psychology of Coaching*. Sydney, Coaching Psychology Unit: University of Sydney.

Griffin, RW (1999) *Management* (6th edition). New York: Houghton Mifflin.

Griffiths, R (1983) *NHS Management Inquiry: Report to the Secretary of State of Social Services*. London: HMSO.

Handy, C (1993) *Understanding Organizations*. London: Penguin.

Hersey, P Blanchard, K and Johnson, D (2007) *Management of Organisational Behaviour* (9th edition). Oxford: Pearson Education.

Herzberg, F (1959) *The Motivation to Work*. New York: John Wiley and Sons.

Hewison, A and Sim, J (1998) Managing Interprofessional Working: Using Codes of Ethics as a Foundation. *Journal of Interprofessional Care*, 12 (3): 309–21.

Hocking, BA (2006) Using Reflection to Resolve Conflict. *Journal of the Association of Operating Room Nurses*, 84 (2): 249–59.

Homans, GC (1961) *Social Behavior: Its Elementary Forms*. New York: Harcourt Brace.

Hopson, B and Adams, J (1976) *Transition: Understanding and Managing Personal Change*. London: Martin Robertson.

House, RJ (2004) *Culture, Leadership, and Organizations: The GLOBE Study of 62 Societies*. Thousand Oaks: Sage.

Howatson-Jones, L (2004) The Servant Leader. *Nursing Management*, 11 (3): 20–24.

International Council of Nurses (2004) *Guidelines on the Nurse Entre/Intrapreneur Providing Nursing Service*. Geneva: ICN Publications. Available online at: www.crnns.ca/documents/Self%20Emp%20Practice/ Guidelines%20for%20Nurse%20Entrepreneurs%20(ICN).pdf.

Jackson, C and Ellis, P (2010) Creative Thinking for Whole Systems Working, in Standing, M (ed) *Clinical Judgement and Decision Making in Nursing and Interprofessional Healthcare* (pages 54–79). Maidenhead: Open University Press.

Janis, IL (1972) *Victims of Groupthink*. New York: Houghton Mifflin.

Janis, IL (1982) *Groupthink: Psychological Studies of Policy Decisions and Fiascos* (2nd edition). New York: Houghton Mifflin.

Johnson, M (1994) Conflict and Nursing Professionalization, in McCloskey, J and Grace, H (eds) *Current Issues in Nursing* (4th edition) (pages 643–9). St Louis: Mosby.

Kotter, J (1990) *A Force for Change: How Leadership Differs from Management*. New York: Free Press.

Kramer, RM, Brewer, B and Hanna, B (1995) Collective Trust and Collective Action: The Decision to Trust as a Social Decision, in Kramer, RM and Tyler, TR (eds) *Trust in Organizations: Frontiers of Theory and Research* (pages 357–89). Thousand Oaks, CA: Sage.

Lawton, A (1998) *Ethical Management for the Public Services*. Open University Press: Buckingham.

Lee, P, Gillespie, N, Mann, L and Wearing, A (2010) Leadership and Trust: Their Effect on Knowledge Sharing and Team Performance. *Management Learning*, 41(4): 473–91.

Lewin, K (1951) *Field Theory in Social Sciences*. New York: Harper and Row.

Linder, D and Ledlow, S (1999) *Five Issues to Be Considered in Teambuilding*. Arizona State University. Available online at: http://clte.asu.edu/active/fiveissues.pdf (accessed 14 October 2010).

Luft, J and Ingham, H (1955) *The Johari Window, a Graphic Model of Interpersonal Awareness*. Proceedings of the Western Training Laboratory in Group Development. Los Angeles: UCLA.

Machell, S, Gough, P and Steward, K (2009) *From Ward to Board: Identifying Good Practice in the Business of the Caring*. London: King's Fund Publications.

Machell, S, Gough, P, Naylor, D, Nath, V, Steward, S and Williams, S (2010) *Putting Quality in the Boardroom*. London: King's Fund Publications.

Mahoney, J (2001) Leadership Skills for the 21st Century. *Journal of Nursing Management*, 9 (5): 269–71.

Marquis, BL and Huston, CJ (2009) *Leadership Roles and Management Functions in Nursing: Theory and Applications*. Philadelphia, PA: Lippincott, Williams and Wilkins.

Maslach, C. (2003) Job Burnout: New Directions in Research and Intervention. *Current Directions in Psychological Science*, 12 (5): 189–92.

Mayer, JD and Salovey, P (1993) The Intelligence of Emotional Intelligence. *Intelligence*, 17(4): 433–42.

Mintzberg, H (1975) *The Manager's Job: Folklore and Fact*. Harvard Business Review, July/August: 66–75.

Mumford, A (1999) *Effective Learning*. London: Chartered Institute of Personnel Development.

NHS Employers (2006) *NHS Employers Guidance – Bullying and Harassment*. London: NHS Employers.

Northam, S (2009a) Conflict in the Workplace: Part 1. Sex, Age, Hierarchy, and Culture Influence the Nursing Environment. *American Journal of Nursing*, 109 (6): 70–3.

Northam, S (2009b) Conflict in the Workplace: Part 2. Strategies to Resolve Conflict and Restore Collegial Working Relationships. *American Journal of Nursing*, 109 (7): 65–7.

Nursing and Midwifery Council (2002) *Supporting Nurses and Midwives through Lifelong Learning*. London: NMC.

Nursing and Midwifery Council (2008) *The Code: Standards of Conduct, Performance and Nursing and Ethics for Nurses and Midwives*. London: NMC.

Nursing and Midwifery Council (2010) *Standards for Pre-registration Nursing Education*. London: NMC.

Nursing Standard (1985) Editorial: First nurses appointed DHA general managers. *Nursing Standard*, 385 (21 February): 1.

Olson, EE and Eoyang, GH (2001) *Facilitating Organization Change: Lessons from Complexity Science*. San Francisco: Josey Bass/Pfeiffer.

Parsloe, E and Leedham, M (2009) *Coaching and Mentoring: Practical Conversations to Improve Learning*. London: Kogan Page.

Pascale, R (1990) *Managing on the Edge*. London: Penguin.

Patterson, C (2005) *Generational Diversity: Implications for Consultation and Teamwork*. Paper presented at the meeting of the Council of Directors of School Psychology Programs on generational differences. Deerfield Beach, Florida.

Quinn, F (1995) *Principles and Practice of Nurse Education*. London: Chapman Hall.

Redshaw, G (2008) Improving the Performance Appraisal System for Nurses. *Nursing Times*, 104 (18): 30–1. Available online at: www.nursingtimes.net/nursing-practice-clinical-research/improving-the-performance-appraisal-system-for-nurses/1314790.article.

SanFacon, G (2008) *A Conscious Person's Guide to the Workplace*. Bloomington: Trafford Publishing.

Scholtes, PR (1998) *The Leader's Handbook: A Guide to Inspiring Your People and Managing the Daily Workflow*. New York: McGraw-Hill.

Schuetze, H and Inman, P (2010) *The Community Engagement and Service Mission of Universities.* Leicester: National Institute of Adult and Continuing Education (NIACE).

Senge, P (1990) *The Fifth Discipline: The Art and Practice of the Learning Organization.* New York: Doubleday.

Senge, P (1996) Leading Learning Organizations. *Training and Development*, 50 (12): 36–34.

Simpson, A (2007) The Impact of Team Processes on Psychiatric Case Management. *Journal of Advanced Nursing*, 60 (4): 409–18.

Smola, KW and Sutton, CD (2002) Generational Differences in Working Age Women. *Journal of Organizational Behavior*, 23 (4): 363–82.

Spouse, J (2001) Work-based Learning in Health Care Environments. *Nurse Education in Practice*, 1: 12–18.

Sullivan, EJ and Decker, PJ (2009) *Effective Leadership and Management in Nursing* (7th edition). Harlow: Pearson International Edition.

Swansburg, RC and Swansburg, RJ (2002) *Introduction to Management and Leadership for Nurse Managers* (3rd edition). Boston: Jones and Bartlett.

The Work Foundation (2005) *Case example.* Available online at: www.theworkfoundation.com/Assets/Docs/Publications/GoodHopeHospital.pdf.

The Work Foundation (2008) *Work-life Balance.* Available online at: www.theworkfoundation.com/research/health/worklifebalance.aspx (accessed January 2011).

Thomas, J (2006) *Survival Guide for Ward Managers, Sisters and Charge Nurses.* London: Churchill Livingstone, Elsevier.

Thomas, KW and Kilmann, RH (1974) *Thomas-Kilmann Conflict Mode Instrument.* Sterling Forest, New York: Xicom.

von Bertalanffy, L (1968) *General System Theory: Foundations, Developments, Applications.* New York: Braziller.

Ward, A (2003) Managing the Team, in Seden, J and Reynolds, J (eds) *Managing Care in Practice* (pages 33–56). London: Routledge.

Williams, J (2007) Follow the Leader. *Healthcare Financial Management*, 61 (1): 50–5.

Wright, P (1996) *Managerial Leadership.* London: Routledge.

Yoder-Wise, P (2007) *Leading and Managing in Nursing* (4th edition). Amsterdam: Elsevier.

Zafirovski, M (2005) Social Exchange Theory under Scrutiny: A Positive Critique of its Economic-Behaviorist Formulations. *Electronic Journal of Sociology.* Available online at: www.sociology.org/content/2005/tier2/SETheory.pdf (accessed 14 December 2010).

Index

Note: Page number in *italics* refers to figures, illustrations, and tables.

A

accommodating, approach for managing conflict situations *65*
Adair, John
    action-centred leadership 100, 145
    ten principles of good time management 145–6
Adams, J. 140–1
Agenda for Change (AfC) bands 41, *41–2*, 113
Antai-Otong, D. 30

B

Bach, S. 49
background information, method for gathering 29
Belbin, Meredith 26–7
Bennis, W.G. 90
Bersin, J. 127
Big Five Personality Theory *see* Five Factor Model of Personality
binary identity 61
binary thinking 61
Bray, L. 78
Bridges, W. 139
    model of transition 139–40
burnout 83

C

care co-ordination 35
Causer, G. 137–8
change theory 114–15, *115–16*, 117
chaos theory 114, 117–18
Chartered Institute of Personnel and Development (CIPD) 62, 111
clinical setting
    bullying in 62–3 *see also* conflict management and negotiation skills
    understanding of the context 7–10
clinical supervision 80
    advantages and disadvantages *86*
coaching
    activities 75, 77
    case example 75
    'GROW' technique 76
    Hersey and Blanchard model 73, *74*

leadership styles for 74
notion of 73–4
three-dimensional (3D) technique 76–7
useful websites for 87
collaboration 35, *64*
communication, in team
    dealing with meetings and committees 31–2
    3 Ps (Preparation, Place and time, and Participation) for meetings 32
    working within professional group/disciplinary group 33–4
competition *65*
complexity theory 114, 117–18
compromising *64*
conceptual feedback loop scheme (Homans) 27, *28*
conflict management and negotiation skills
    activities 60–1, 63, 65–6
    approaches to managing conflict *64–5*, 64–9
    arbitration/conciliation, use of 67
    case example 57–8
    identifying sources of conflict 60–3
    importance in care environments 58–60
    in learning organisations 64
    management of yourself and your relationships 68–9
    mediation, use of 66–7
    negotiation, use of 66
    strategies to prevent conflict 63–4
    understanding conflict 57–8
    whistle blowing 67–8
consensus, importance in culturally diverse society 31, 49, 67
cultural dimensions, in workplace 48–9

D

Daft, R. 90
decision making, effective *24*
Decker, P.J. 25, 29
delegation of tasks, in team 40–1
    activities 41
    enabling staff development through 43–4
directness, importance in culturally diverse society 49
discussion, effective *24*
dodging, strategy for conflict management *65*

E

emotional intelligence 65, 69, 97, 149
   case example 101
   development of 149
   Goleman's framework 101
   role of 101–2
entrepreneur 93, 119
entrepreneurship 119–20
environment, effective *24*
Eoyang, G.H. 117
Equality Act (2006) 59
Essential Skills Clusters (ESCs) 2, 37, 55–6, 72,
    88, 105, 124–5, 136
Exworthy, M. 137–8

F

feedback, effective 23, *24*
feelings, effective *24*
Five Factor Model of Personality 47–8
Foundation Trusts 110–11
freedom of choice 28

G

Gallway, Tim 76
Gantt Chart 115
good leader/manager
   characteristics 12–13
   examples of 12–13
   preparing for a leadership or management
     role 142–9
   see also leadership and management
governance 31, 106, 109–17, 120
Grant, A. 49
Griffin, R.W. 94
group dynamics 21–2
   see also team(s)
group think 32
   symptoms of 33

H

Handy, Charles 14
Hawthorne effect 94
Health and Safety at Work Act (1974) 59
healthcare assistants (HCAs)
   Associate Practitioner (AP) roles 41
   job description (JD) *41–2*
   National Vocational Qualifications (NVQs)
     42–3
   Qualifications Credit Framework (QCF)
     42
Hewison, A. 34

hierarchy, importance in culturally diverse
   society 49
Holmes–Rahe Life Event Rating Scale 141
Homans, George 27
   conceptual feedback loop scheme 27, *28*
Hopson, B. 140
Human Rights Act (1998) 113
Huston, C. J. 111

I

individualism, importance in culturally diverse
   society 49
individuals in team
   appraisal in nursing 45–7
   baby boomers 49–51
   decision making 41
   delegation 40–1
   developmental level of individuals *44*
   generational differences 49–51
   gen Xers 49–51
   and individual differences 47
   individual roles, responsibility, and
     accountability 38–40
   millennials 49–51
   organisational culture 48–9
   personal development plans 44–5
   skill mix 41–3
   staff development 43–4
   traditionalists 49–51
   useful websites for 53–4
information sharing 35, 93, 144
Ingham, Harry 11
integrity 13, 18–19, 77, 147
intelligence 12
   social 69
   see also emotional intelligence
interdisciplinary team working 33–4
   activities 34
intergenerational conflict and team work
    49–51
International Council of Nurses (ICN) 119
interprofessional working, effective 34

J

Janis, Irving 32
Johari window 11, *11*, 127
   blind area 11
   hidden area 11
   open/free area 11
   unknown area 11

K

Knowledge Skills Framework website 44
Kotter, J. 44, 73

L

leader, effective 10
leadership and management
    activities 39, 91, 95, 97, 99–100, 139, 141,
        146–7, 149
    approach to 1
    Bridges' model of transition *139–40*
    context of values for 6
    debate 89–91
    differences between managers and leaders 90
    Hopson and Adams model of transition to
        leadership *140–1*
    importance 1
    for individuals in team *44*
    policy context 17
    preparing for a leadership or management
        role 142–9
    self esteem and transition 139–42
    stages from practice to management *137–8*
    theories of leadership 98–102
    theories of management 91–5
    transition to leadership 137–42
    understanding of the context 7–10
    understanding ourselves and other's
        perception 11–12
    useful websites for 104, 150
leadership/management role, preparing for
    142–9
    Adair's ten principles of good time
        management 145–6
    effective communication 144
    effective listening 144
    emotional intelligence, developing 149
    learning from mistakes 145
    motivation development 142–3
    resilience, developing 147–9
    self belief 144–5
    sorting of challenging situation 148–9
    understanding values 147
leadership, theories of
    Adair's action-centred leadership 100
    emotional intelligence, role of 101–2
    gaining support, role of 102, *102*
    person-centred nature of health and social
        care 101
    servant leader 100–1
    transactional leadership 98

transformational leadership 98–9
learning cultures 73, 81, 85, 127–31
learning environment
    activities 126, 128
    of care 126–7
    definition 127
    developing 132–4
    elements of 129–31
    importance of 128–9
    NMC Standard of proficiency 132
    perspective of the ward manager 129
    project management template for *134*
    Senge's model *130*
    useful websites 135
learning organisation 80–2
    activities 82
    features of 82
learning styles, useful websites for 86
Lee, P. 127
legitimate power 14–15
Lewin, Kurt 114–15, 117
listening, effective 51, 66, 144
Local Health Watch organisations 111
Lorenz, Edward 118
Luft, Joseph 11

M

McLennan, M. 115–16
management, theories of
    contingency theory 93–4
    Mintzberg's role theory 92–3
    resilience 96–7
    systems theory 94–5
    workload management 95–6
manager, effective 10, *24*
Marquis, B.L. 111
mediation 55, 66–7
mental health nurses 43, 83
mentoring
    activities 78
    buddying schemes 79
    vs. coaching 77
    in healthcare settings 79
    historical relevance 77
    multi-professional views of 78–9
    NMC standards 77–8
    notion of 73–4
    useful websites for 87
Mid Staffordshire Hospitals 13
Mintzberg, H. 144
    role theory 92–3, 95

moral management 96
Motivation–Hygiene theory of job satisfaction *142–3*
multi-disciplinary mental health team 34

N
National Institute for Health and Clinical
  Excellence (NICE) 17, 111
National Service Frameworks (NSFs) 17
negative/destructive criticism 23
Nettleton, P. 78
nurse entrepreneur 119
nurse intrapreneur 119
nurse leadership, structures of 14–17
  activities 16
  case example 16
  legitimate power 14–15
  managerial power and responsibility 14
  non-managers function as leaders 15
  Nursing and Midwifery Council (NMC), role
    of 17
  useful websites 19
nursing, team problems in 30
Nursing and Midwifery Council (NMC)
  Code of Professional Conduct (2008) 17, 38
  competencies for nurses 2, 55, 72, 88, 105,
    124, 136
  standard of proficiency for learning
    environment 132
  Standards Domain Leadership 34
  Standards for Pre-registration Nursing
    Education 2–3, 5, 20, 37–8, 55, 72, 88,
    105, 124, 136

O
Olson, E.E. 117
organisational aspects of care
  Agenda for Change (AfC) pay agreement 113
  case examples 110
  change management 113–20
  governance arrangements 109–13
  management by objectives (MBO) 112
  nurses at Board level, role of 108–9
  organisational structures 107–8
  peer review process 112
  performance management 111–12
  reward schemes 113
  understanding the organisation 106–7
  useful websites 123
organisational culture 48–9
  activities 48
othering 61

P
Pascale, R. 90
Patterson, C. 49, 51
performance appraisal 111–13, *121–2*
  individuals in team 45–7
personal accountability 30
personal development plan (PDP) 44–5
Post Registration Education and Practice
    (PREP) 45
Princes' Youth Business Trust 79
psychiatric case management, team processes
    on 34–5
Public Information Disclosures Act (1998) 68

Q
Quinn, F. 127

R
Redshaw, G. 45–6
refreezing 114–17
resilience 96–7
  developing 148–9
response, effective *24, 33*

S
SanFacon, G. 145
Scholtes, P.R. 102
Senge, Peter 130
Sim, J. 34
skill mix 41–3, 81, 96
Smola, K.W. 50
social capital 65
social exchange theory 27–8
social intelligence 69
social networking site 50
social obligations 28
span of control 107
Spouse, J. 128
stakeholders 115–16
Sullivan, E.J. 25, 29
Sutton, C.D. 50

T
tasks/responsibilities, effective *24*
team building, aims of 29
team(s)
  activities 21–2
  communication in 31
  dealing with meetings and committees 31–2
  definition 22
  developing effective 29–30

effectiveness 22–4
facilitating team think 32–3
giving constructive feedback 23–4
group dynamics 21–2
helpful team activity dealing differences 23
influence of social system on 27
norms 25
nurturing roles *26*
preliminary preparation for a team building
    exercise 29
professional codes of conduct 23
3 Ps (Preparation, Place and time, and
    Participation) for meetings 32
psychiatric case management, team processes
    on 34–5
questions related to characteristics of an
    effective team 29–30
roles 25–7
strategies for managing problems of 30
team problems in nursing 30
uncomfortable situations to deal within 23
useful websites for building and managing
    36
water cycle analogy 27
working within professional group or
    disciplinary 33–4
team think, concept of 32–3
total quality management 58
Traynor, M. 119

U
UK community mental health teams 34–5
understanding the context 7–10
    about integrity 13
    activities 9–12
    enduring difficulties for student nurses 7–8
    inability and its consequences 7
    methods 9
    perceptions and knowledge about ourselves
        and shared by others 11–12
    as quality of a good manager or leader 8
United Kingdom Council for Nursing and
    Midwifery 80
unrefreezing 114, *115*

V
values 147
    about leadership and management 6
    of practising nurses 9
Von Bertalanffy, L. 94

W
water cycle analogy 27
whistle blowing 34, 67–8
Williams, J. 142
work-life balance 83–5
    useful websites for 87
workload management 95–6